How to Pivot from Burnout to Balance

The 7-Step Science-Backed System to Recharge Your Energy, Reduce Stress and Thrive—Without Overhauling Your Life

By Andrea Sinclair

© Copyright Andrea Sinclair 2025 - All rights reserved.

The content contained within this book may not be reproduced, duplicated or transmitted without direct written permission from the author or the publisher.

Under no circumstances will any blame or legal responsibility be held against the publisher, or author, for any damages, reparation, or monetary loss due to the information contained within this book. Either directly or indirectly. You are responsible for your own choices, actions, and results.

Legal Notice:

This book is copyright protected. This book is only for personal use. You cannot amend, distribute, sell, use, quote or paraphrase any part, or the content within this book, without the consent of the author or publisher.

Disclaimer Notice:

Please note the information contained within this document is for educational and entertainment purposes only. All effort has been executed to present accurate, up to date, and reliable, complete information. No warranties of any kind are declared or implied. Readers acknowledge that the author is not engaging in the rendering of legal, financial, medical or professional advice. The content within this book has been derived from various sources. Please consult a licensed professional before attempting any techniques outlined in this book.

By reading this document, the reader agrees that under no circumstances is the author responsible for any losses, direct or indirect, which are incurred as a result of the use of the information contained within this document, including, but not limited to, — errors, omissions, or inaccuracies.

ISBN (Paperback): 978-1-0692940-7-4
ISBN (Hardcover): 978-1-0692940-8-1
ISBN (eBook): 978-1-0692940-6-7

Table of Contents

YOU DESERVE BETTER—AND IT STARTS TODAY ------ 7

CHAPTER 1: UNDERSTANDING BURNOUT—THE SILENT ENERGY KILLER -- 9

CHAPTER 2: THE BURNOUT RECOVERY MINDSET—REWIRING HOW YOU APPROACH STRESS ------------- 19

CHAPTER 3: THE ENERGY RESET—HOW TO RECHARGE PHYSICALLY AND MENTALLY ------------------------------ 33

CHAPTER 4: BOUNDARIES THAT STICK—PROTECTING YOUR ENERGY WITHOUT GUILT ------------------------- 53

CHAPTER 5: MENTAL RESILIENCE—REWIRING YOUR MIND TO HANDLE STRESS BETTER ---------------------- 79

CHAPTER 6: PURPOSE AND MEANING—HOW TO REIGNITE MOTIVATION AND JOY ----------------------------------- 102

CHAPTER 7: SUSTAINABLE HABITS—HOW TO PREVENT BURNOUT FROM COMING BACK ----------------------- 120

CHAPTER 8: THE 7-STEP BURNOUT RECOVERY PLAN—YOUR PERSONALIZED BLUEPRINT FOR BALANCE - 136

YOUR PATH TO A BURNOUT-FREE LIFE -------------- 154

I BELIEVE IN YOU --- 157

A HEARTFELT THANK YOU ------------------------------ **157**

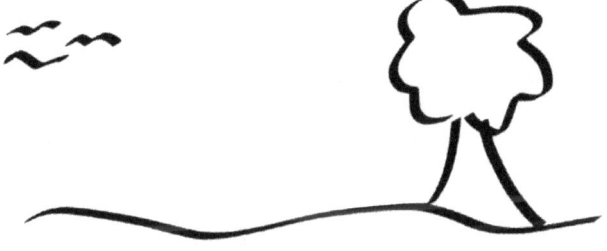

A Free Thank You Gift

As a token of my appreciation and a way of saying thanks for your purchase, I'm offering the short book **Sleep Your Way to Balance: Nighttime Rituals to Recharge Your Body and Mind** for FREE to my readers.

To get instant access scan the QR code or just go to:

https://andreasinclairbooks.com/free-gift

Inside the book, you will discover:

- Nighttime Rituals to Recharge
- Science-backed Tips and Tricks
- 30 Minute Wind Down Formula

If you want to improve your sleep and feel better, make sure to grab the free book!

You Deserve Better—And It Starts Today

"You didn't wake up burned out one morning—it happened gradually. But now, you're stuck in a cycle where rest doesn't feel like rest and motivation is nowhere to be found."

Burnout isn't just about feeling tired—it's about reaching a point where your body, mind, and spirit feel depleted, leaving you stuck in a cycle of exhaustion and overwhelm. It creeps in slowly, disguised as dedication, ambition, and the desire to keep up. You tell yourself to push through, to just get to the weekend, the vacation, the next milestone—but the exhaustion doesn't go away. It lingers, seeping into every aspect of your life, until you no longer recognize the vibrant, driven person you used to be.

I know this feeling all too well. For years, I lived in a constant state of overdrive—late nights, endless to-do lists, and the ever-present pressure to do more, be more. I told myself it was just a rough season, that things would ease up soon. But the truth was, my body had been sending distress signals for months—headaches, brain fog, restless sleep. I ignored them. Until one morning, I found myself sitting in my car in the office parking lot, too drained to walk inside. I had nothing left to give. That moment was my wake-up call. I realized burnout wasn't a badge of honor—it was a warning sign that something had to change.

That realization set me on a journey to uncover what truly works to reverse burnout—not just temporary fixes, but sustainable, science-backed strategies that restore energy, reduce stress, and bring real balance. I dove into the research, consulted experts, and tested every method myself. What I discovered is that reclaiming your energy doesn't require overhauling your entire life. It's about making small but powerful shifts that lead to big results.

This book is your guide to that transformation. In the next chapters, I'll walk you through a 7-step system designed to help you break free from burnout, recharge your mind and body, and find balance—without quitting your job, uprooting your life, or adding more to your already full plate. These are strategies grounded in neuroscience, psychology, and the lived experiences of people who have successfully made the shift.

If you're here, it means you're ready for change. And I want you to know: sustainable balance is possible. By the time you turn the last page, you'll have a clear roadmap to regain your energy, set healthy boundaries, and feel like yourself again.

It's time to take back control. Let's begin.

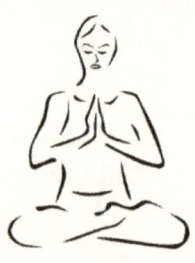

Chapter 1

Understanding Burnout—The Silent Energy Killer

"Burnout isn't just exhaustion—it's a full-system shutdown. If you've ever felt like you're running on empty, you're not alone. Nearly 77% of professionals say they've experienced burnout at work, and the consequences affect every area of life—your health, relationships, and happiness."

1.1 What Burnout Really Is (and What It's Not)

Burnout is not just an extension of stress—it's something far more profound. Stress is a natural response to pressure, and when managed properly, it can even enhance performance. Burnout, on the other hand, is a state of complete mental, physical, and emotional depletion. It doesn't just make you feel exhausted—it changes the way you think, work, and engage with life. Unlike stress, which often has a clear cause and a temporary duration, burnout builds over time and doesn't go away with a good night's sleep or a weekend off.

The Three Stages of Burnout

Burnout doesn't happen overnight. It develops in stages, with warning signs along the way:

1. The Honeymoon Phase: High energy and commitment drive you to push harder, but small signs of fatigue or frustration begin to appear.
2. Chronic Stress: You start feeling overwhelmed more frequently, experience disrupted sleep, and rely on caffeine, sugar, or other quick fixes to power through.
3. Burnout: At this stage, exhaustion becomes the norm. Motivation plummets, mental clarity fades, and even small tasks feel insurmountable.

Recognizing these stages early is critical to preventing total burnout. The sooner you acknowledge the warning signs, the easier it is to reverse course and restore balance before reaching full depletion.

Why Willpower Alone Won't Fix It

Many people assume they can push through burnout with sheer determination. But burnout isn't about a lack of willpower—it's a biological and psychological response to prolonged stress. Chronic stress rewires your brain, depletes key neurotransmitters, and disrupts your body's ability to recover. Simply deciding to "try harder" won't solve the problem because burnout affects your ability to make decisions, regulate emotions, and sustain motivation.

The key to overcoming burnout is not to push through—it's to step back, reassess, and implement proven strategies that support both your brain and body. That's exactly what this book will help you do.

Now that you understand what burnout really is, let's explore the first step in reclaiming your energy and balance.

1.2 The Science of Burnout: What's Happening in Your Brain and Body

Burnout isn't just a mindset—it's a physiological state that affects your entire nervous system. When stress becomes chronic, it alters your brain chemistry, drains your energy reserves, and leaves you feeling physically and mentally depleted. To break free, you need to understand what's happening inside your body.

The Cortisol Trap: How Chronic Stress Rewires Your Nervous System

When you're under constant stress, your body stays in a prolonged state of fight-or-flight mode, flooding your system with cortisol. In small doses, cortisol helps you stay alert and focused, but chronic stress keeps these levels elevated, leading to fatigue, anxiety, and even memory problems. Over time, your nervous system becomes dysregulated, making it harder to relax, sleep, or feel energized, even when you're not actively stressed.

Decision Fatigue and Cognitive Overload: Why You Feel Drained Even Doing Simple Tasks

Have you ever felt exhausted by the end of the day, even if you didn't do anything particularly demanding? That's decision fatigue at work. Your brain can only make so many choices before it starts to slow down, making even simple decisions feel overwhelming. Burnout magnifies this effect, reducing your ability to concentrate, problem-solve, and think creatively. It's why even routine tasks, like answering emails or deciding what to eat for dinner, can feel exhausting when you're burned out.

Your Body's Warning Signals: Hidden Burnout Symptoms Most People Ignore

Burnout doesn't always show up as sheer exhaustion right away. Your body sends warning signals, but they're often dismissed as minor inconveniences. Some common but overlooked symptoms include:

- Persistent headaches or muscle tension
- Digestive issues, such as bloating or nausea
- Frequent colds or weakened immunity
- Feeling emotionally detached or irritable
- Difficulty sleeping, even when exhausted

Recognizing these signals early can help you take action before burnout reaches a breaking point. In the next chapter, we'll explore how to shift from burnout to balance using simple, science-backed strategies that restore your energy and resilience.

1.3 Identifying Your Burnout Type

Burnout isn't one-size-fits-all. It wears different masks, sneaks into our lives in different ways, and affects us based on our unique responsibilities, personalities, and stressors. The first step toward reclaiming your energy and balance is recognizing the specific burnout pattern that has taken hold of your life.

The Overachiever's Burnout: When Perfectionism Leads to Exhaustion

You're driven, ambitious, and capable—but at what cost? If you constantly push yourself to hit impossible standards, work long hours, and say yes to everything, you might be suffering from Overachiever's Burnout. It's fueled by perfectionism, an inner critic that tells you rest is a weakness, and a relentless cycle of doing more to prove your worth. The result? You're exhausted, overwhelmed, and no matter how much you accomplish, it never feels like enough.

The truth: You don't need to burn out to succeed. In fact, success and sustainability go hand in hand. The key is learning to redefine achievement—not as constant hustling, but as meaningful, focused progress that includes rest and recovery.

The Caregiver's Burnout: When Giving Too Much Leaves You Depleted

You take care of everyone—your family, your colleagues, your community—but who takes care of you? Caregiver's Burnout happens when you pour so much of yourself into others that there's nothing left in your own tank. Whether you're a parent, a healthcare professional, a leader, or simply the one everyone turns to, this burnout sneaks in when your generosity becomes self-sacrifice.

The truth: Giving doesn't have to mean depletion. Boundaries, self-care, and asking for help aren't selfish—they're necessary. The strongest caregivers are the ones who understand that their well-being matters too.

The Boredom Burnout: When Work Drains You Because It Lacks Meaning

Burnout isn't always about working too hard—it can also be about not feeling connected to what you do. If your days feel monotonous, uninspiring, or like you're just going through the motions, you may be experiencing Boredom Burnout. This type of exhaustion stems from disengagement rather than overwork, leaving you drained, unmotivated, and questioning, Is this all there is?

The truth: Purpose is the antidote to burnout. It doesn't mean you have to quit your job or overhaul your life overnight. Small shifts—aligning your work with your values, seeking new challenges, or carving out time for passion projects—can reignite your energy and sense of fulfillment.

Your Burnout Type Is Your Starting Point

Recognizing which burnout pattern resonates with you most is the first step toward recovery. Burnout isn't a personal failure—it's a signal that something needs to change. The good news? You can make that change. And it doesn't require a dramatic life overhaul—just intentional shifts that will help you recharge, realign, and thrive.

Your Chapter 1 Challenge: The Burnout Awareness & Action Challenge

After reading through the first chapter and understanding what burnout truly is, what it looks like in different forms, and how it impacts both your brain and body, it's time to take a moment for self-reflection and action. This challenge is designed to help you identify your current burnout type and begin the process of recognizing how burnout is manifesting in your life. By the end of this exercise, you'll have a clearer understanding of where you stand and a small first step toward recovery.

Step 1: Identify Your Burnout Type

Take a few minutes to reflect on the different burnout types outlined in Section 1.3. Which of the following best describes your current experience?

- The Overachiever's Burnout: Do you constantly strive for perfection, feeling like nothing is ever good enough? Are you pushing yourself harder and harder, yet still feeling drained, with little to show for it?

- The Caregiver's Burnout: Do you find yourself overwhelmed by the needs of others, often sacrificing your own well-being in the process? Are you stretched thin by trying to help everyone, leaving yourself with little to no energy for yourself?

- **The Boredom Burnout:** Does your work feel uninspiring, draining, and lacking in meaning? Do you feel mentally and emotionally exhausted because your work no longer excites you, leaving you stuck in a cycle of disengagement?

Once you've identified your burnout type, take a moment to acknowledge how this is impacting your daily life. Are there specific situations or patterns that trigger these feelings?

Step 2: Track Your Energy Levels

For the next 3 days, track your energy levels throughout the day. Use the following scale to rate how you're feeling:

- 0-2: Extremely drained, exhausted, or overwhelmed.
- 3-5: Tired, but functional; could use a break.
- 6-8: Generally energized, but with some fatigue.
- 9-10: High energy, feeling great.

At each major point in your day (e.g., morning, mid-day, and evening), make a note of how you're feeling and what you were doing at the time. Did a specific task, interaction, or environment contribute to a drop in energy? Did you feel better when you took a break or engaged in a restorative activity?

Step 3: Spot Your Triggers

Based on your energy tracking, take a look for patterns and triggers. Are there particular activities or stressors that seem to drain you more than others? For example:

- Is it the constant need to perform at a high level (Overachiever's Burnout)?
- Are you putting others' needs before your own to the point where you have nothing left (Caregiver's Burnout)?
- Or do you feel bored and disengaged in your daily tasks, leading to a sense of emptiness (Boredom Burnout)?

Write down your most significant triggers. This exercise will help you build self-awareness, so you can begin taking intentional steps to address them.

Step 4: Commit to One Small Change

Now that you have identified your burnout type and potential triggers, choose one small action to reduce the impact of burnout in your life. Here are some ideas based on the burnout types:

- For Overachievers: Set a boundary today by saying "no" to one task or responsibility you feel you're pushing yourself to do. Let go of the perfectionism and focus on progress over perfection.

- For Caregivers: Schedule 30 minutes of personal time each day to recharge. This could be a walk, a hobby, or simply sitting in silence. Remember, your needs are just as important as others'.

- For the Bored: Find one task or project that feels meaningful to you, even if it's just a small aspect of your work or life. Commit to engaging in it fully for at least 15 minutes today. A sense of purpose can help combat burnout.

Set a timer for yourself, and make this small change today. It might be uncomfortable at first, but even these incremental shifts will start to make a big difference in how you approach burnout.

Reflection: At the end of the week, take a moment to reflect on what you've learned from this challenge. Do you feel more aware of your burnout triggers? Did the small change you made create any noticeable shifts in your energy levels or mindset? Share your thoughts and progress in a journal or with a supportive friend. This self-awareness is the first crucial step toward shifting from burnout to balance.

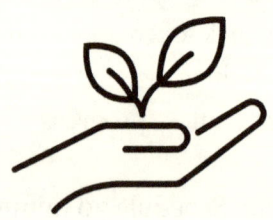

Chapter 2

The Burnout Recovery Mindset—Rewiring How You Approach Stress

"You can't fix burnout with the same mindset that caused it. Recovery starts by changing how you think about work, rest, and self-worth."

2.1 Reframing Productivity—Why Working Less Can Make You Achieve More

In a world that glorifies hustle culture, we're constantly bombarded with the message that more hours worked equals more success. We've been conditioned to believe that pushing ourselves to the limit is the only path to achievement. But what if the very thing we think is helping us move forward is actually holding us back?

The Myth of Hustle Culture: How Overwork is Sabotaging Your Success

For decades, we've been taught that success requires sacrifice—long hours, sleepless nights, constant stress. In fact, hustle culture has become a badge of honor. We wear our exhaustion like a trophy, convincing ourselves that being constantly busy means we're moving closer to our goals. But this myth is not only unhealthy; it's counterproductive.

Overwork breeds burnout, and burnout leads to mental and physical exhaustion, reduced creativity, and diminished focus. The more we push ourselves, the less we can accomplish. It's time to challenge the belief that "hustle" is synonymous with "success" and embrace a new mindset—one where working smarter, not harder, is the key to achieving your dreams.

The Law of Diminishing Returns: Why Working More Hours Doesn't Mean Getting More Done

The Law of Diminishing Returns states that after a certain point, the more effort you put into a task, the less effective your results become. In simple terms: working longer hours doesn't equal more output. In fact, it often leads to decreased productivity and creativity.

When you're tired, stressed, and overwhelmed, your ability to focus and perform at your best diminishes. It's like trying to run on a flat tire—no matter how hard you push, you're going nowhere fast. Instead of pushing through exhaustion, it's essential to recognize the point at which the returns on your time start to shrink and give yourself permission to stop, recharge, and come back stronger.

Energy vs. Time Management: The Secret to Getting More Done While Doing Less

If you want to truly get ahead, it's not about managing your time better—it's about managing your energy. Time is a finite resource, but energy is something we can replenish, refocus, and direct. While time is always ticking away, your energy is what fuels your work and enables you to perform at your best.

Rather than fixating on squeezing more tasks into your schedule, prioritize activities that help you recharge, whether it's a quick walk, meditation, or simply getting enough sleep. By optimizing your energy, you'll find yourself not only more productive but more present and creative in every area of your life.

The truth is, you don't have to work yourself into the ground to succeed. It's time to let go of the hustle myth and embrace a new approach: work less, but work smarter. When you prioritize energy over time, you'll achieve more with less effort, and in the process, reclaim your balance and your joy.

2.2 The Power of Micro-Shifts in Recovery

When you're burnt out, the idea of making drastic changes can feel overwhelming—almost impossible. The truth is, the road to recovery doesn't have to be a monumental overhaul. In fact, the most powerful shifts often come in the form of small, consistent changes. These micro-shifts, though seemingly insignificant, have the power to create profound transformation when practiced over time. Let's explore how these subtle adjustments can lead to a more balanced, energized life.

The 1% Rule: Why Small Changes Have the Biggest Impact Over Time

The key to lasting change isn't about making grand, sweeping gestures. It's about committing to small, incremental improvements—just 1% better every day. This is the core principle behind the 1% Rule. Small changes, practiced consistently, compound over time and create a ripple effect in all areas of your life.

Think of it this way: if you improve by 1% every day, within a year, you'll have improved by 37 times. That's a massive shift, but it doesn't require monumental effort. Whether it's drinking an extra glass of water, taking a 5-minute mindfulness break, or getting an extra hour of sleep, these tiny actions add up. You'll begin to see that you don't need to completely overhaul your routine to experience transformation. It's the small wins that build the foundation for big results.

A Short Story: A Single Step Forward

Let me share a personal story that illustrates the power of the 1% Rule.

Several years ago, I found myself completely exhausted and overwhelmed. I had a demanding career, two young kids, and was trying to keep everything together. I was barely keeping my head above water. One day, after yet another sleepless night, I realized something had to change. But I couldn't fathom another major overhaul. The idea of completely reworking my routine felt like more of a burden than a solution.

So, I decided to start small. I began by committing to just one 5-minute meditation every morning before I got out of bed. It wasn't much, but it was something I could manage. Over time, I added more little changes—drinking more water, taking a walk during lunch, turning off email notifications after 7 p.m. None of these actions on their own seemed life-changing, but they began to stack up. Over a few months, I noticed a significant shift in my energy levels, my mindset, and my ability to handle stress. It wasn't a dramatic, all-at-once transformation—but I had made real progress, one tiny step at a time.

The Two-Minute Stress Reset: Simple Ways to Recalibrate Your Nervous System Instantly

When stress hits, it's easy to feel like you're stuck in a never-ending cycle of tension and overwhelm. But what if you could reset your nervous system in just two minutes? The power of micro-shifts lies in their ability to help you recalibrate in the moment, without needing hours of meditation or therapy. Simple, effective practices can break the cycle of stress and return you to a state of balance quickly.

One effective technique is a quick breathing exercise. Inhale deeply for a count of four, hold for four, and exhale slowly for four. Repeat this cycle for two minutes. This activates your parasympathetic nervous system, calming your body's stress response and bringing you back to a state of relaxation. It may seem small, but these short moments of recalibration are powerful enough to interrupt stress patterns and bring you back to your center.

Another easy reset is the "grounding" technique. Simply stand up, take off your shoes, and press your bare feet into the ground for a moment. Focus on the sensations of the earth beneath you. This practice can quickly reconnect you to the present moment, helping you release tension and gain clarity.

From All-or-Nothing to Progress-Oriented Thinking: Why Perfectionism Keeps You Stuck

One of the biggest barriers to recovery and growth is the all-or-nothing mindset. When you feel burned out, it's tempting to think you must either make a complete overhaul of your life or nothing will change. This black-and-white thinking often stems from perfectionism—the belief that if you can't do something perfectly, it's not worth doing at all.

The truth is, perfectionism keeps you stuck in a cycle of inaction and self-criticism. It's not about doing everything flawlessly—it's about making progress, even if that progress is small. Shifting from all-or-nothing thinking to a progress-oriented mindset is one of the most freeing changes you can make. Instead of aiming for perfection, focus on improvement. Every step forward, no matter how small, is a victory. Celebrate those micro-shifts, and remember: it's the little changes that lead to big results.

These micro-shifts are your secret weapons in the battle against burnout. By embracing small changes, resetting your stress in moments, and letting go of perfectionism, you can begin to reclaim your energy and your balance. Progress isn't always about dramatic transformations—it's about making consistent, manageable shifts that, over time, build momentum and lead to profound healing.

2.3 The Science of Rest—Why You're Still Tired Even After Sleeping

It's a familiar scenario: you go to bed exhausted, sleep for a full eight hours (or more), and wake up still feeling tired, foggy, and drained. You might wonder—how is this even possible? If you're getting the recommended amount of sleep, why are you still struggling to feel energized and refreshed?

The answer lies in the fact that true rest goes beyond just sleeping. Your body, mind, and spirit require more than one kind of rest to truly recover. In fact, there are seven different types of rest that are necessary for recharging your energy. Let's explore the science of rest, why sleep alone isn't enough, and how you can start feeling more restored, faster.

The 7 Types of Rest You Actually Need: Why Sleep Alone Isn't Enough

Sleep is crucial to our health, but it's not the only type of rest your body needs to truly recover. Dr. Saundra Dalton-Smith, a physician and rest researcher, identifies seven types of rest that every person needs to thrive:

1. **Physical Rest**
   This type of rest is what most people associate with sleep, but it also includes passive activities like taking naps, using techniques like yoga or stretching, or simply resting without any physical exertion.

2. **Mental Rest**

   Our minds are constantly working, even when we're not consciously aware of it. Mental rest is crucial to give your brain a break from overthinking, problem-solving, or multitasking. Mindful activities such as deep breathing, meditation, or simply taking a break from screens can help.

3. **Sensory Rest**

   In today's world, our senses are constantly bombarded with stimuli—from emails, to social media notifications, to the hustle and bustle of everyday life. Sensory rest involves creating quiet, calm environments to give your eyes, ears, and mind a chance to recover.

4. **Emotional Rest**

   Emotional rest comes from letting go of the constant demands of other people and allowing yourself to feel your emotions without the pressure to "be strong" or "keep it together." Journaling, talking with a supportive friend, or spending time alone can provide emotional rest.

5. **Social Rest**

   We often feel drained not just by the work we do, but by the people we interact with—whether it's clients, coworkers, or even family members. Social rest involves stepping away from people who drain your energy and spending time with those who uplift and support you.

6. **Creative Rest**

   Our creativity needs to be replenished just as much as our energy. If your job or life requires you to be constantly creative—whether it's solving problems, generating ideas, or working in a creative field—then you need creative rest. This could mean taking time off from your usual creative tasks to engage in a completely different activity, like nature walks or practicing a hobby that nurtures your imagination.

7. **Spiritual Rest**

   Spiritual rest involves feeling connected to something greater than yourself—whether it's through religious practices, nature, or personal reflection. When you feel disconnected from your sense of purpose or spirituality, it can drain your energy. Spiritual rest allows you to restore that connection.

As you can see, sleep alone doesn't fulfill all of these needs. Without incorporating all seven types of rest into your life, you may continue to feel drained despite getting plenty of sleep. The key is to intentionally rest in all of these areas to experience true restoration.

Active vs. Passive Rest: How to Restore Energy Faster

Not all rest is created equal. Active rest and passive rest are two distinct approaches, and knowing the difference can help you restore your energy more effectively.

- Passive Rest involves stillness and relaxation, like sleep, meditation, or lying down. This kind of rest is essential for physical recovery and can help your body repair itself after exertion.

- Active Rest, on the other hand, involves moving your body in ways that promote relaxation and energy restoration, such as gentle yoga, walking, or swimming. Active rest is great for increasing circulation, reducing muscle tension, and boosting your overall energy levels without taxing your body.

Incorporating both active and passive rest into your routine allows for quicker and more complete recovery. For instance, after a busy day, a gentle walk can give your mind a break and reduce stress, while a short nap can recharge your physical energy. By balancing these two types of rest, you'll find that your energy is restored more effectively and at a faster pace.

Signs Your "Rest" Habits Are Keeping You Drained: What to Avoid

Just because you're sleeping doesn't mean you're fully resting. In fact, there are common habits that may be keeping you drained, even after a night of sleep. Here are a few signs your rest habits may not be as effective as you think:

How to Pivot from Burnout to Balance

1. **Relying on Screens Before Bed**
   The blue light emitted by phones, tablets, and computers disrupts your natural sleep cycle, making it harder to fall into a deep, restorative sleep. If you're scrolling or watching TV before bed, you're likely not giving your body the chance to fully unwind.

2. **Over-scheduling Rest Time**
   You might be "resting" by binge-watching TV or scrolling through social media—but these activities don't allow for true mental or emotional recovery. Passive entertainment doesn't provide the type of rest your body and mind need to recharge.

3. **Staying Busy During Rest Time**
   If you're constantly multitasking, even when "resting," you may be robbing yourself of true recovery. Checking work emails during downtime or engaging in stimulating conversations can prevent your brain from getting the mental rest it requires.

4. **Ignoring Your Body's Cues**
   If you're always pushing through tiredness or disregarding the need for rest, you're setting yourself up for burnout. Pay attention to the physical and emotional signals your body is sending you—sometimes, your body needs a full break, not just a nap.

The science of rest is clear: sleep alone is not enough to restore your energy. You need a holistic approach, incorporating physical, mental, emotional, and spiritual rest into your daily routine. By understanding the different types of rest and learning how to use both active and passive rest effectively, you can begin to feel more energized, focused, and ready to take on the world.

Your Chapter 2 Challenge: A Seven Day 7 Minute a Day Reset

One of the best ways to improve your rest habits is to make time each day to engage in a quick and effective reset. Here's a simple daily challenge to help you integrate the various types of rest into your routine:

The 7-Minute Rest Reset Challenge:

Each day, set aside 7 minutes to focus on a specific type of rest. For the next week, try the following:

1. **Day 1: Physical Rest (Passive)**
   Take 7 minutes to lie down and do nothing. No screens, no distractions—just focus on letting your body completely relax. You can lie on your back, do some gentle stretching, or just let go of all tension. Use a pillow or bolster for extra comfort.

2. **Day 2: Mental Rest**
   Spend 7 minutes in complete silence, focusing only

on your breath. Inhale deeply for a count of 4, hold for 4, and exhale for 4. If your mind begins to wander, gently bring your attention back to your breath.

3. **Day 3: Sensory Rest**

   Close your eyes, sit in a quiet space, and just listen to the sounds around you. Pay attention to the most subtle sounds—whether it's the hum of the refrigerator, the distant sound of traffic, or the wind rustling the trees outside. For the next 7 minutes, let your senses absorb this peace without interruption.

4. **Day 4: Emotional Rest**

   Take 7 minutes to journal or write down any thoughts or emotions you're currently holding onto. Don't worry about perfection—just express what's on your mind. Let it all out, and then take a moment to sit in stillness and let your emotions be without judgment.

5. **Day 5: Social Rest**

   Disconnect from social media and take 7 minutes to simply sit alone, without any interaction or external influence. This time is for you to recharge away from the social demands of the world.

6. **Day 6: Creative Rest**

   Spend 7 minutes doing something creative that isn't related to your work. It could be doodling, knitting, cooking, or even taking photos. The goal is to engage your creativity in a low-pressure, nonproductive way.

7. **Day 7: Spiritual Rest**
   Take 7 minutes to reflect on something that gives you a sense of peace or purpose. This could be a prayer, a moment of gratitude, a walk in nature, or even just sitting quietly with your thoughts, letting go of stress and reconnecting with what nourishes your soul.

By incorporating this 7-minute rest challenge into your daily routine, you'll begin to address the various dimensions of rest and recharge your body, mind, and spirit more holistically. Even on the busiest of days, carving out just 7 minutes can help you reclaim your energy and restore your balance.

Chapter 3

The Energy Reset—How to Recharge Physically and Mentally

"If your phone ran out of battery as often as you do, you'd replace the charger. It's time to find what actually recharges you."

3.1 Eating for Energy Instead of Exhaustion

When you're burned out, your energy feels like it's constantly on a rollercoaster ride—up one moment, crashing down the next. And while it's easy to blame lack of sleep, the truth is that the food you eat plays a significant role in either fueling your body for recovery or keeping you stuck in a cycle of exhaustion. The way we nourish ourselves can either support a balanced energy system or add to the fuel of burnout.

In this section, we'll dive into how your diet can either lift you up or drag you down, and how small adjustments can make a significant difference in your energy levels, mood, and ability to handle stress.

The Blood Sugar Rollercoaster: How Food Affects Fatigue

One of the biggest culprits behind fatigue is a lack of stable blood sugar. When you eat foods that cause your blood sugar to spike and crash, you're essentially creating a rollercoaster of energy throughout the day.

Here's how it works:
When you consume refined carbs (think sugary snacks, white bread, pastries) or sugary drinks, your blood sugar rises rapidly. This quick surge can give you a burst of energy, but it's short-lived. Your body responds by releasing insulin to lower your blood sugar. This often results in a "crash" as your energy levels dip, leaving you feeling fatigued, irritable, or unfocused.

This cycle of blood sugar highs and lows is exhausting, and it's a major contributor to burnout. The constant energy fluctuations make it harder to feel consistently energized and focused, and can leave you reaching for caffeine or another sugar boost to get through the afternoon.

The Solution? Eat foods that stabilize your blood sugar. Focus on incorporating fiber-rich foods (like vegetables, whole grains, and legumes) and lean proteins (like chicken, fish, or tofu). These foods digest more slowly, releasing energy over a longer period of time and keeping you feeling sustained and balanced.

Burnout-Proof Nutrition: Easy Food Swaps to Sustain Energy

Nutrition doesn't have to be complicated, and you don't need to make drastic changes to start feeling better. A few simple swaps can help you avoid the blood sugar rollercoaster and sustain your energy throughout the day:

1. Swap refined carbs for grains:
   Instead of white bread or pasta, opt for whole grains like quinoa, brown rice, or oats. These complex carbohydrates release energy more slowly, keeping your blood sugar steady and preventing that dreaded energy crash.

2. Add healthy fats to your meals:
   Healthy fats, such as those from avocados, nuts, seeds, and olive oil, provide long-lasting energy and help you feel full longer. They also support brain health, which can help improve focus and clarity during burnout recovery.

3. Eat protein with every meal:
   Protein helps stabilize blood sugar and supports muscle repair. Include lean protein sources like eggs, turkey, fish, or plant-based options like lentils and chickpeas in your meals to keep your energy levels steady throughout the day.

4. Snack smart:
   Instead of reaching for sugary snacks, opt for combinations that include both protein and fiber, like a handful of nuts with some fruit, or hummus with vegetables. This will help maintain your energy without the inevitable crash.

5. **Hydrate with water, not sugary drinks:** Dehydration can contribute to fatigue, so it's important to drink plenty of water throughout the day. If you're craving something with flavor, try infusing your water with fruits or herbs like lemon, cucumber, or mint for a refreshing twist.

Caffeine and Burnout: When Coffee Helps and When It Makes Things Worse

Ah, caffeine—the magical elixir that keeps many of us going, especially when burnout makes us feel like we're running on empty. While coffee or tea can offer a temporary energy boost, it can also make things worse in the long run, especially if you're relying on it to power through exhaustion.

Here's the catch:
Caffeine works by stimulating your central nervous system, giving you a quick boost of alertness and energy. However, when consumed in excess or at the wrong time, caffeine can disrupt your sleep patterns, heighten anxiety, and leave you feeling more tired once the effects wear off. For people dealing with burnout, caffeine can become a crutch, leading to a vicious cycle of reliance and energy crashes.

So, how can you tell if caffeine is helping or hurting your burnout recovery? Here are some key points to consider:

- **When Coffee Helps:**
  If you enjoy your morning cup of coffee and it helps you feel more alert, it can be a useful tool in

moderation. Just be mindful of your caffeine intake and avoid drinking it late in the day, as it can interfere with your sleep.

- **When Coffee Makes It Worse:**
  If you find yourself reaching for caffeine multiple times a day to stay awake, it could be a sign that your body is already too fatigued and your reliance on coffee is only masking the deeper issue. In this case, it's time to reconsider how much caffeine you're consuming and explore other energy-boosting methods, like better sleep, hydration, or nutrition.

One strategy is to slowly reduce your caffeine intake while increasing your intake of water, herbal teas, or other natural energy sources. Aim to drink your coffee earlier in the day and avoid it after 2 p.m. to prevent disrupting your sleep. Slowly tapering your caffeine use can help reset your body's natural energy rhythms.

Eating for energy isn't about restrictive dieting or cutting out your favorite foods entirely—it's about making smart food choices that help stabilize your blood sugar, nourish your body, and keep your energy levels consistent throughout the day. By swapping out processed foods for whole, nutrient-dense options and being mindful of your caffeine habits, you can start fueling your body for recovery rather than contributing to your exhaustion.

3.2 Movement as Medicine

When you're burned out, the last thing you may feel like doing is exercising. The idea of "moving more" can sound exhausting, especially when you're already running on empty. However, what if I told you that smart, intentional movement could actually be one of the most powerful tools in your recovery toolkit? Exercise doesn't have to be about "more" or pushing yourself to the limit—it's about "better" and finding ways to move that energize and restore you, not drain you further.

In this section, we'll explore how the right kind of movement can fuel your energy, improve your mood, and even help you recover faster from burnout.

Why Exercise Isn't About "More" But "Better": Smart Movement for Energy

When we're in a state of burnout, we're often conditioned to think that we need to push through and do more to feel better. This mindset can be particularly harmful when it comes to exercise. We may feel like we need to follow extreme workout routines or push ourselves into intense cardio sessions to "burn off" stress or fatigue. But the truth is, when we're already depleted, this kind of "more is better" mentality can backfire.

Instead of focusing on how much you're doing, think about what you're doing—and why. The key to recovery is choosing forms of movement that are restorative, efficient, and energizing. You don't need to run a marathon or spend hours at the gym. Instead, aim for smart movement that supports your body's natural rhythms, provides stress relief, and recharges your energy reserves.

The Anti-Burnout Workout: Quick, Effective Ways to Boost Energy

When you're in recovery mode from burnout, you need workouts that help to activate your body in a way that doesn't leave you feeling wiped out afterward. The Anti-Burnout Workout is all about quick, energizing movement that focuses on recovery rather than exertion.

Here are some effective anti-burnout exercises that require little time but can provide significant benefits:

1. Gentle Yoga or Stretching (10-15 minutes)
   Yoga is a great way to release built-up tension, stretch tight muscles, and calm the nervous system. Focus on gentle flows or restorative poses that help you reconnect with your body and breath. Even just 10 minutes can leave you feeling more grounded and relaxed.

2. Walking (15-20 minutes)
   Walking is one of the most underrated forms of exercise. It's simple, accessible, and has been shown to boost mood, improve circulation, and reduce stress. A brisk walk around the block, or in a nearby park, can provide a significant energy boost, without draining you.

3. Bodyweight Strength Training (10 minutes)
   Strength training doesn't have to mean lifting heavy weights. Simple bodyweight exercises like squats, lunges, or push-ups can activate your muscles, promote circulation, and leave you feeling stronger and more energized. Focus on low-impact movements, and go for a shorter, more efficient session rather than a long, strenuous one.

4. Breathing Exercises (5-10 minutes)
   Deep breathing exercises can actually energize you and reduce the physical symptoms of stress. Try a technique like box breathing (inhale for 4 seconds, hold for 4 seconds, exhale for 4 seconds, hold for 4 seconds), or diaphragmatic breathing, to activate your parasympathetic nervous system, reduce anxiety, and restore focus.

By incorporating these short but effective workouts, you can begin to reclaim your energy without feeling the need to push yourself beyond your limits. The goal is to move with intention and focus on how your body feels—energized, restored, and grounded—not exhausted and depleted.

Movement Breaks vs. Exercise: When You Don't Have Time for a Full Workout

We've all had those days where the thought of squeezing in a full workout feels impossible. Between meetings, family obligations, and general life chaos, finding time for long exercise sessions can feel like a luxury. But even on your busiest days, movement is still possible—and can be incredibly beneficial.

Incorporating movement breaks throughout the day is a great way to combat burnout and stay energized, even when time is tight. Movement breaks are short, intentional bursts of activity that can break up your workday, improve circulation, and reduce mental fatigue. Here are some simple ways to get your body moving:

1. Stretching Break (2-5 minutes)
   Stand up, stretch your arms above your head, and reach for the sky. Stretch your back, shoulders, and legs. This can help relieve tension and prevent stiffness from sitting too long, boosting your mood and energy.

2. Walk or Stand (5-10 minutes)
   If you've been sitting for a long period, take a quick walk around the house or office, or stand up and move around while you work. Even just 5 minutes of walking can improve circulation and refresh your mind.

3. Chair Exercises (2-3 minutes)
   If you're tied to your desk, try seated exercises like seated leg raises or seated torso twists. These low-impact movements will help activate your muscles without needing to leave your workspace.

4. Dance Party (2-3 minutes)
   This one's fun: Put on your favorite song and dance

around for a couple of minutes. It's a great way to get your blood flowing, shift your mood, and add some joy to your day—all in a short time.

The beauty of movement breaks is that you don't need to set aside a significant block of time to experience the benefits. A few minutes here and there can go a long way in reducing stress, boosting energy, and supporting your recovery from burnout.

Movement for a Balanced Life

The truth is, exercise doesn't have to be about doing more; it's about doing better. By incorporating smart, effective movement into your routine—whether through quick workouts or simple movement breaks—you can start to experience the restorative benefits of movement without adding extra strain on your body. Prioritize movement that supports your energy, rather than drains it, and make it an essential part of your burnout recovery.

3.3 The Sleep Fix—Rebuilding Your Energy Bank

Sleep is the ultimate remedy when it comes to burnout recovery—but what happens when you wake up feeling just as exhausted as you did when you went to bed? The problem might not be that you're not sleeping enough, but rather that the sleep you're getting isn't quality sleep. If your sleep patterns are disrupted or misaligned with your body's natural rhythm, it's like trying to deposit energy into an overdrawn bank account—you never feel fully recharged.

In this section, we'll explore why burnout causes sleep problems, how to reset your natural sleep rhythms, and what pre-bedtime habits can help you relax and actually get the restorative rest you need.

The Burnout Sleep Pattern: Why You Wake Up Exhausted

One of the most frustrating aspects of burnout is that, no matter how much sleep you get, you often wake up feeling worse than when you went to bed. This is a common symptom of burnout, and it stems from a combination of factors that affect the quality of your sleep.

- Chronic Stress and Elevated Cortisol: Burnout is deeply linked with chronic stress, which leads to elevated levels of cortisol (the stress hormone) in the body. Cortisol should naturally decline in the evening to help you wind down, but when you're burned out, cortisol levels can remain high, making it difficult for your body to relax and sleep deeply.

- Sleep Disruption from Overstimulation: Many people who are burned out struggle with overstimulation—whether it's mental (thinking about work) or physical (screen time late at night). This can disrupt your body's natural sleep cycle, preventing you from falling into the deep, restorative stages of sleep.

- Restlessness and Nighttime Anxiety: Burnout often brings with it a cycle of anxiety, racing thoughts, or a constant "to-do" list running in the background. This mental chatter can interfere with your ability to get restful sleep, leaving you feeling mentally and physically drained the next day.

The solution isn't simply to sleep longer—it's to focus on quality sleep. This means addressing the factors that are preventing you from achieving restful, deep sleep.

The 90-Minute Rule for Better Sleep: How to Reset Your Natural Rhythm

Did you know that your body operates on a natural 90-minute sleep cycle? Every 90 minutes, you pass through different stages of sleep—from light sleep to deep, restorative sleep, followed by REM (Rapid Eye Movement) sleep, which is crucial for memory and emotional regulation. The problem is, if your sleep cycle is disrupted—whether by stress, late-night habits, or inconsistent sleep patterns—you're not allowing your body to complete these cycles properly, which results in waking up feeling groggy, unrested, and unrefreshed.

The 90-minute rule is a simple concept: aim to wake up at the end of a complete 90-minute sleep cycle, rather than in the middle of one. This can help you feel more rested and less groggy upon waking.

Here's how it works:

- Set a sleep goal based on 90-minute cycles. For example, if you want to get 7.5 hours of sleep, you'll want to aim for 5 full 90-minute cycles. This would mean going to bed at a time that allows you to wake up at the end of a cycle—such as 10:30 p.m. to wake up at 6 a.m.
- Experiment with your sleep time to find the sweet spot for your body's rhythm. You can try adjusting your bedtime to see when you feel most rested after waking up.

While it may take some trial and error to find your ideal sleep cycle, using the 90-minute rule can help you align your sleep with your body's natural rhythms and improve the quality of your rest. You'll wake up feeling more refreshed and energized, and your body will be better equipped to handle the stresses of the day.

How to Wind Down When You're Too Stressed to Sleep: Effective Pre-Bedtime Habits

One of the most common challenges of burnout is being too stressed to sleep. When your mind is racing with thoughts about work, life, or what you didn't get done today, it's difficult to wind down. But establishing a pre-bedtime routine can signal to your brain that it's time to shift into relaxation mode, even on your most stressful days.

Here are some simple but powerful habits to incorporate into your evening routine:

1. **Ditch the Screens 30-60 Minutes Before Bed:**
Blue light from phones, tablets, and computers disrupts your body's production of melatonin, the hormone that helps you sleep. Make it a habit to stop using screens at least 30 minutes before bedtime. Instead, engage in calming activities like reading, journaling, or listening to soothing music.

2. **Establish a Relaxing Ritual:**
Create a calming pre-bedtime ritual that signals to your body it's time to wind down. This could include:

    - Gentle stretching or yoga to release muscle tension.
    - A warm bath or shower to relax your body.
    - A cup of herbal tea like chamomile or lavender, which have natural sedative properties.

3. **Practice Mindfulness or Meditation:**
Taking a few minutes to meditate or practice deep breathing can help calm your mind and prepare you for sleep. Progressive muscle relaxation is a great technique: starting from your toes and working your way up, tense each muscle group for a few seconds, then release. This can help ease both physical and mental tension.

4. **Journal Your Thoughts:**
If your mind is racing with worries, take a few minutes to write them down. Journaling can help you release anxious thoughts and prevent them from

lingering in your mind. Write down a "brain dump" of everything on your mind or jot down three things you're grateful for—it helps shift your focus and calm your mind.

5. **Limit Stimulants After Midday:**
   As discussed in the previous section, caffeine can disrupt sleep if consumed too late. Make sure to avoid caffeine in the afternoon and evening to give your body enough time to wind down naturally.

By incorporating these habits into your routine, you'll gradually train your body to relax and prepare for deep, restorative sleep. The goal is not only to get enough sleep but to improve the quality of the sleep you're getting, so that you wake up feeling genuinely rested, instead of dragging yourself through the day.

Rebuilding Your Energy Bank

Burnout depletes your energy reserves, but quality sleep is the most powerful way to restore them. By following the 90-minute rule and creating a calming pre-bedtime routine, you can retrain your body's natural sleep cycles and wake up feeling revitalized, not exhausted. The key is consistency and creating habits that help signal to your body that it's time to unwind, relax, and recharge.

Your Chapter 3 Challenge: Rebuild Your Energy and Boost Your Recovery

Now that you've learned about the powerful connection between nutrition, movement, and sleep in your burnout recovery, it's time to put that knowledge into action. This challenge is designed to help you restore your energy, reduce stress, and begin feeling more balanced. For the next 7 days, try the following steps:

Day 1: Balance Your Energy with Food

- Action: Take note of how you feel throughout the day based on what you eat. Focus on stabilizing your blood sugar by eating small meals that include protein, fiber, and healthy fats. Aim to swap out refined sugars for whole grains, lean protein, and veggies.
- Goal: By the end of the day, notice if your energy feels more consistent, and avoid those mid-afternoon crashes.

Day 2: Movement for Energy

- Action: Start with a 10-minute walk or light stretching session. If you're up for it, try a 10-minute bodyweight workout that includes squats, lunges, or gentle yoga stretches. Pay attention to how your body feels before and after moving.
- Goal: Focus on intentional movement that restores, not exhausts, your energy. Notice if it lifts your mood or helps you feel less tense.

Day 3: Prioritize Sleep with the 90-Minute Rule

- Action: Go to bed at a time that allows you to wake up at the end of a 90-minute sleep cycle. For example, if you need to wake up at 6:30 a.m., aim to go to sleep by 10:30 p.m. Adjust your bedtime by 90-minute intervals for optimal rest.
- Goal: Set an intention to wake up feeling more refreshed and rested. Track how much more energy you have throughout the next day.

Day 4: Pre-Bedtime Wind-Down Routine

- Action: Create a 30-minute wind-down routine that includes activities like reading, stretching, or practicing deep breathing. Try a guided meditation or progressive muscle relaxation to help you unwind.
- Goal: Ensure your pre-bedtime routine is screen-free and soothing. Notice if you fall asleep more easily and wake up feeling less anxious.

Day 5: Movement Breaks for Energy Boosts

- Action: Set a timer for a movement break every 2-3 hours. Stand up, stretch, walk around, or do a 2-minute dance party. See how it impacts your focus and energy.
- Goal: Notice how taking movement breaks helps reduce physical and mental fatigue. This is a great way to avoid feeling drained after sitting for long periods.

Day 6: Experiment with Nutrition Timing

- Action: Eat a balanced breakfast and try not to skip meals. Consider adding healthy fats (like avocado or nuts) and protein (like eggs or plant-based options) to sustain you. Have a lighter, easily digestible meal for dinner.
- Goal: Observe how your energy levels are impacted by the timing of your meals and how they keep your blood sugar levels more stable throughout the day.

Day 7: Reflect and Re-Evaluate

- Action: Take some time to reflect on your week. How do you feel physically, emotionally, and mentally? Have you noticed any positive shifts in your energy, stress levels, or sleep quality? What habits worked best for you, and which ones would you like to continue?
- Goal: Write down three things you can continue doing to sustain your progress. Remember, small changes add up over time.

Bonus Tip: If you want to make this challenge even more personalized, jot down one thing you'll commit to adding each week for the next month, based on the habits that resonated with you the most.

This challenge is designed to be actionable, achievable, and grounded in science, focusing on small, consistent changes that will build a foundation for long-term recovery from burnout. Keep track of your progress, and don't be too hard on yourself if you miss a day—it's about progress, not perfection.

You've got this! Let's get started.

Chapter 4

Boundaries That Stick—Protecting Your Energy Without Guilt

"Burnout isn't just caused by doing too much—it's caused by saying 'yes' too much. Let's fix that."

4.1 The Art of Saying No Without Feeling Bad

Saying "no" might feel like a minor word, but for many of us, it holds immense power—power that often feels uncomfortable, guilt-laden, or even confrontational. We live in a culture that values productivity, people-pleasing, and saying yes to every opportunity, request, or responsibility that comes our way. But here's the truth: saying yes to everything is a fast track to burnout. And unfortunately, it's also a surefire way to disregard your own needs.

In this section, we'll explore why saying "no" can be so difficult, and more importantly, how you can do it without guilt or overthinking. By mastering the art of saying no, you'll not only protect your time and energy but also take back control of your life.

Why You Feel Guilty Setting Boundaries: The Psychology Behind It

For many people, saying "no" triggers a sense of guilt. It feels wrong, selfish, or like we're letting others down. This guilt can be rooted in a few key psychological factors:

- Fear of Disappointing Others: We may fear that saying no will lead to others being disappointed in us, angry with us, or thinking we're not "good enough." It's natural to want to be liked and accepted, and saying no can feel like we're putting up a wall between ourselves and others.

- People-Pleasing Conditioning: If you've spent a lifetime putting others' needs first, you may have developed a habit of prioritizing their requests over your own. This can feel virtuous on the surface, but it leaves you drained and stretched too thin.

- Overvaluing Responsibility: Many people struggle with saying no because they feel an overwhelming sense of responsibility. We think if we don't step up, no one else will, and things will fall apart. But here's the hard truth: overcommitting only leads to burnout, and no one can be everything to everyone all the time.

- Perfectionism: If you're someone who thrives on "doing it all," saying no can feel like admitting failure or imperfection. But in reality, perfectionism is often the enemy of progress. You can't do everything, and trying to leads to mental and physical exhaustion.

The good news is that guilt around saying no is something you can learn to manage. The key is to reframe your mindset and understand that setting boundaries is not selfish—it's self-care.

Scripts for Saying No Gracefully: How to Decline Requests with Confidence

Mastering the art of saying no is all about having the right mindset and the right words. Here are some simple, effective scripts you can use to decline requests confidently and without guilt:

1. The Direct Approach

    - "Thank you for thinking of me, but I'm unable to take on any additional commitments right now."
    - "I've got a lot on my plate at the moment, so I'm going to have to pass."

2. The Apology-Free Approach

    - "I'm focusing on my well-being right now, so I need to decline this time."
    - "I've been prioritizing some personal projects, so I can't commit to this."

3. The Offer to Help in a Different Way

- "I can't take on this task, but I'd be happy to help you brainstorm or point you in the right direction."
- "While I can't participate, I'd be glad to offer advice or resources that may help."

4. The "Maybe Later" Approach

- "That sounds interesting, but I'm not able to take it on right now. Let's touch base in a few months to see if I can help."
- "I'm tied up at the moment, but I'll reach out if I have availability in the future."

The key is to be firm but polite, and avoid over-explaining or justifying your decision. Saying no doesn't require a long list of excuses—it simply requires honesty and self-respect.

The 24-Hour Rule: How to Break the Habit of Overcommitting

One of the most powerful tools in your arsenal for saying no is the 24-hour rule. This simple strategy allows you to pause and reflect before making commitments, preventing you from jumping into obligations without consideration. The 24-hour rule works like this:

- When a request is made (whether it's for a meeting, a favor, or a new project), take 24 hours before responding. This gives you time to think about whether you truly have the energy, time, and capacity to say yes. It also gives you the opportunity to assess whether this request aligns with your priorities and boundaries.

- If the request is urgent, explain that you need a moment to evaluate. You can say something like: "Let me take 24 hours to consider this, and I'll get back to you."

- In those 24 hours, consider the following:

    - Do you genuinely have the capacity to take this on?
    - Does this align with your current priorities?
    - Will saying yes take you away from more important tasks or self-care?

By giving yourself this breathing room, you reduce the pressure to make snap decisions. Often, after 24 hours, the urgency fades, and you can say no without guilt or hesitation.

Practice Saying No—It's a Skill

Saying no is a skill that takes practice. In fact, it's a skill you can refine over time. Here are some tips to help make it easier:

- Start small: Begin by saying no to less important requests. For example, decline an invitation to an event you don't feel like attending or turn down a task at work that someone else can handle. The more you practice, the more comfortable you'll get with saying no in larger situations.

- Role-play: If you struggle with saying no, practice with a friend or in front of the mirror. The more you say it out loud, the more confident you'll become when the time comes.

- Be compassionate with yourself: It's okay to feel guilty in the beginning. Practice self-compassion and remind yourself that saying no is an act of self-preservation. Your boundaries are an important part of maintaining your energy, well-being, and peace of mind.

The Takeaway

Learning to say no without guilt is an essential part of overcoming burnout and taking back control of your time and energy. By understanding the psychology behind why we feel guilty and using practical strategies like clear scripts and the 24-hour rule, you can begin setting healthy boundaries with confidence. Remember: Saying no is not a rejection of others—it's a declaration of your commitment to your own well-being.

Example: Setting Boundaries at Work

Scenario:

Samantha, a working mother and manager at a marketing

firm, is feeling overwhelmed with the demands of her job and personal life. She's been asked by her boss to take on a new project that would require extra hours and weekend work. Samantha's already struggling to balance her existing workload with caring for her children, and she knows that taking on this new project will only push her closer to burnout.

Before Setting Boundaries:
Samantha feels guilty about saying no. She worries that her boss will think she's not committed to her career or that she'll let the team down. She also doesn't want to disappoint anyone or appear incapable of handling her responsibilities.

Using the 24-Hour Rule:
Instead of immediately agreeing or feeling pressured, Samantha tells her boss, "Thank you for thinking of me for this project. It sounds like an important initiative, but I'm going to need to take 24 hours to evaluate my current workload before I can confirm whether I can take it on."

This gives Samantha the time to assess her priorities and consider whether this new project fits with her boundaries.

After 24 Hours:
After some reflection, Samantha realizes that taking on this project would negatively affect her family time and increase her stress levels. She also knows that her mental and physical health is more important than stretching herself too thin at work.

Saying No Gracefully:
The next day, Samantha sends her boss the following message:

"After giving it some thought, I've realized I'm unable to take on this project due to my current workload and personal commitments. I believe it would be unfair to both the team and myself if I were to take it on right now. I would be happy to revisit it in the future or assist in finding someone else who may have the capacity to take it on."

Outcome:
Her boss appreciates her honesty and understands her situation. Samantha has set a clear boundary and doesn't feel overwhelmed or guilty, as she took the time to consider her limits first. She's also able to focus on her priorities—her health, family, and existing projects.

Lesson:
In this situation, Samantha's decision to pause and think through her response using the 24-hour rule helped her avoid overcommitting. By politely saying no, she was able to protect her time and energy, and she didn't sacrifice her well-being in the process. Instead of feeling guilty, she now feels empowered and more in control of her life.

This example shows how you can use the strategies of the 24-hour rule and graceful scripts to say no, set boundaries, and protect your energy, even in work situations where the pressure to say yes is high. Does this example feel aligned with what you had in mind? Would you like me to adjust any details?

4.2 Work Boundaries That Keep Burnout Away

In today's world, work often spills over into every aspect of our lives. The rise of technology, remote work, and the constant demand for instant replies has blurred the lines between work and personal time. But here's the hard truth: not creating boundaries between work and life is one of the most common causes of burnout. Whether you're working from the office or remotely, it's crucial to establish clear work boundaries that allow you to recharge, protect your well-being, and stay energized for both your professional and personal life. In this section, we'll dive into practical strategies to create boundaries that keep burnout at bay and help you maintain a healthier, more balanced life.

How to Stop Working After Work: Creating Clear Mental Separation

When you're deep into a busy workweek, it's easy to let work consume your time, energy, and even your thoughts long after you've clocked out. The constant "just one more email" mentality can make it difficult to switch off. But if you want to prevent burnout, it's essential to create a clear mental separation between work and your personal life.

Here are some actionable strategies to stop working after hours and truly disconnect:

1. Set a Firm "End of Day" Time:
   Decide on a specific time each day that marks the end of your workday. It could be 5 p.m. or 7 p.m. depending on your schedule. Once that time hits,

close your laptop, turn off work notifications, and put your phone out of sight. It's important to set this boundary and stick to it, even if it feels uncomfortable at first.

2. Create a Physical Workspace Separation (if you work from home):
    If you're working remotely, the line between home and office can get very blurry. Create a designated workspace that you only use during working hours. Once the workday is over, physically leave that space—go for a walk, spend time with family, or relax in a different area of your home. This physical separation will help your mind distinguish between "work mode" and "off time."

3. Implement a "Transition Ritual":
    Create a simple ritual that signals the end of your workday. It could be something as simple as closing your computer, making a cup of tea, or journaling for a few minutes. This transition helps your mind shift from work mode to relaxation mode. Over time, your brain will associate this ritual with rest, making it easier to unwind.

4. Set Boundaries with Family/Household Members:
    When you're home, it's easy to fall into the trap of being "always on" for family or household tasks as well. Set clear expectations with your loved ones about when you are and aren't available to help with errands, chores, or other demands.

Just as you set work boundaries, it's essential to set personal boundaries.

How to Handle a Boss Who Expects 24/7 Availability: Proven Strategies

With many workplaces adopting a 24/7 work culture and using digital tools to stay connected, it's no surprise that some bosses expect constant availability. However, this expectation can lead to exhaustion, burnout, and loss of personal time. If you're dealing with a boss who expects you to be available around the clock, it's essential to take charge of the situation and set boundaries that protect your time and energy.

Here are some strategies to handle a boss who expects 24/7 availability:

1. **Communicate Your Work Hours Clearly:** One of the most important steps is to clearly communicate your working hours to your boss and colleagues. For example, you can say, "My working hours are from 9 a.m. to 6 p.m., and I'll be available for work-related matters during that time. After hours, I make it a point to disconnect so I can recharge for the next day." This sets a firm but polite expectation and helps others understand your boundaries.

2. **Set Expectations Around Urgency:** Let your boss know how to determine when

something truly needs your attention after hours. For example, you can explain, "I'm happy to address urgent matters after hours, but I ask that non-urgent issues be saved for the next day." This establishes a clearer distinction between things that require immediate attention and those that can wait.

3. **Use "Do Not Disturb" Settings and Notifications:**

   In today's digital world, work messages can come through at any time of day. Use technology to your advantage by setting "Do Not Disturb" notifications on your phone and email after hours. This lets your boss (and colleagues) know that you're offline, without having to respond immediately.

4. **Lead by Example:**

   If your boss is setting unrealistic expectations of availability, be proactive in leading by example. Show how you manage your time effectively during working hours and deliver high-quality work within those parameters. Over time, your boss will come to respect your boundaries and might even set similar expectations for the team.

Remote Work Burnout: Avoiding the "Always-On" Trap

Remote work has its perks: no commute, more flexibility, and the comfort of home. But it also comes with its own set of challenges, including the "always-on" mentality. When you're working from home, it's easy to slip into the habit of constantly checking your email, responding to Slack messages late into the evening, or simply being "on" all the time. This lack of separation between work and life is a breeding ground for burnout.

Here are strategies to avoid remote work burnout and create better boundaries:

1. **Set Specific Work Hours:**
   Establish clear working hours, just as you would if you were in a traditional office setting. If you start work at 9 a.m., make sure you finish by 5 p.m. (or whatever works for your schedule). Stick to your work hours, and resist the temptation to check in on work outside of those times.

2. **Designate a "Work Zone":**
   If possible, create a dedicated workspace in your home—preferably in a room with a door you can close at the end of the day. If you don't have a separate room, a corner of a room or a desk can work too. This helps mentally separate work from personal life.

3. **Take Frequent Breaks:**
   Incorporate regular breaks into your day. Get up, stretch, go for a walk, or do something non-work-related every 90 minutes. Breaks help you maintain focus and energy throughout the day, preventing burnout from prolonged sitting and work without respite.

4. **Use Technology Mindfully:**
   Technology is both a gift and a curse in remote work. Set boundaries on your phone and email, and consider using apps that remind you to take breaks or that block work-related notifications after hours. Additionally, set aside time for non-work activities, like family time, hobbies, or exercise, and commit to staying off work platforms during those moments.

5. **Plan Downtime:**
   In remote work, it's easy to overwork and forget to prioritize rest. Schedule regular downtime during your week where work is completely off-limits. This downtime allows you to recharge and return to work with renewed energy and focus.

The Takeaway

Creating and maintaining work boundaries is critical for avoiding burnout and staying balanced. By setting firm limits around your work hours, communicating expectations with your boss, and actively managing your availability (especially in remote work environments), you can take back control of your time. Remember: setting boundaries isn't about rejecting others—it's about preserving your energy and well-being for the long term. Your personal life and health matter just as much as your professional success.

4.3 Emotional Boundaries—Protecting Yourself from Draining Relationships

We all have relationships that vary in their emotional energy output. Some relationships are nourishing, uplifting, and leave you feeling energized, while others—often without you realizing it—can leave you feeling drained, depleted, or even emotionally exhausted. These are the relationships you need to protect yourself from, the ones that might leave you feeling like you're constantly giving without getting anything back. They can sometimes be called energy vampires—individuals who, consciously or unconsciously, drain your emotional and mental energy.

Establishing emotional boundaries is one of the most important steps in protecting your well-being and preventing burnout. In this section, we'll explore how to set limits with draining people, how to prioritize your own needs without feeling guilty, and how to figure out how much socializing is enough for you to maintain your balance.

How to Deal with Energy Vampires: Setting Limits with Draining People

Energy vampires can come in many forms: they could be well-meaning friends, family members, colleagues, or even acquaintances who constantly demand your time, emotional support, or attention. They tend to focus on their own needs or problems without recognizing the toll it takes on you.

The key to dealing with these energy-draining relationships is to set firm emotional boundaries. Here's how:

1. Recognize the Signs:
   Before you can set a boundary, it's important to recognize when someone is draining your energy. Pay attention to how you feel after spending time with certain people. Do you feel emotionally exhausted, anxious, or resentful? If so, it's time to evaluate the relationship and identify whether this person is an "energy vampire."

2. Identify the Cause:
   Often, energy vampires aren't intentionally trying to deplete your energy. Many times, they may be seeking validation, empathy, or support that they need. Understanding the root cause of their behavior can help you approach the situation with empathy while still setting boundaries that protect your energy.

3. Set Clear Limits:
   Be firm but compassionate. You don't have to say "no" in an aggressive or harsh way, but you can set limits. For example, if a friend constantly vents about their problems without reciprocating, you could say:

   - "I understand you're going through a lot right now, but I'm feeling a bit overwhelmed myself. Can we talk about something more uplifting or lighter today?"
   - "I'm happy to listen, but I can't continue this conversation right now. Let's pick it up another time when I'm able to be fully present."

4. Practice Self-Awareness:
   Recognize when a person is pulling you into their emotional storm, and give yourself permission to disengage. You're allowed to step back from a conversation if it's too draining. This can be as simple as gently excusing yourself or redirecting the conversation to a different topic.

5. Communicate Your Needs:
   Let people know what you need in a respectful way. It could be as simple as saying, "I need some quiet time this evening to recharge" or "I'm feeling too tired to have a long conversation today." It's okay to prioritize your own emotional health.

The Guilt-Free Guide to Prioritizing Yourself: Letting Go of People-Pleasing

One of the greatest challenges in setting emotional boundaries is the guilt that often accompanies saying "no" or prioritizing your own needs over others. People-pleasing behaviors can drain your energy and contribute to burnout, but letting go of this need to constantly please others is essential for your emotional well-being.

Here's how you can prioritize yourself guilt-free:

1. **Understand Your Own Needs:**
   The first step to letting go of people-pleasing is understanding that you have needs, too. Just because someone asks something of you doesn't mean you are

obligated to comply, especially if it's at the cost of your own well-being. Start by checking in with yourself regularly: "Do I really have the energy for this? Is this in alignment with my own priorities?"

2. **Practice Saying No with Kindness:**
   Saying no doesn't have to mean rejecting someone or being rude. It can simply mean protecting your own boundaries. A simple, kind refusal could be:

   - "I'd love to help, but I need to take care of myself today."
   - "I'm unable to commit to that right now, but thank you for thinking of me."

3. **Reframe the Word "No":**
   Instead of seeing "no" as a rejection, reframe it as a positive declaration of your own needs. Saying no to one thing often means saying yes to something better for you—whether that's rest, personal time, or focusing on something more important.

4. **Recognize the Impact of Overcommitment:**
   Over-committing to others often means you're not able to show up fully for yourself or for those who truly matter. When you feel the urge to please, take a moment to think about how saying yes will impact your energy, your mental health, and your well-being in the long run. Saying no allows you to show up in a more meaningful and authentic way in the relationships that truly matter.

5. **Seek Support When Needed:**
   If you find it difficult to let go of people-pleasing tendencies, it may be helpful to work with a therapist or coach to dig into the underlying causes of this pattern. Understanding why you feel the need to please others can help you shift your mindset and build healthier habits.

The Power of "Minimum Effective Dose" in Socializing: How Much Is Enough?

Another important aspect of maintaining emotional boundaries is figuring out how much socializing is enough for you. For some people, socializing can be energizing, while for others, it can be draining. The concept of "Minimum Effective Dose" (MED)—a term borrowed from the world of health and fitness—refers to the smallest amount of something you need to experience the benefits without overdoing it.

When it comes to socializing, you don't have to attend every party, meet every friend, or answer every message. Understanding your MED of social interaction is crucial to avoid burnout and protect your emotional energy.

Here are some tips for practicing the MED principle in socializing:

1. Know Your Limits:
   Pay attention to how you feel after social events. Do you feel energized and connected, or drained and tired? If socializing starts to feel like a chore, it may

be a sign that you're overextending yourself. Understanding when you've reached your socializing limit will help you avoid burning out.

2. Schedule Downtime After Socializing:
If you know you have a busy week of social events ahead, make sure you schedule some recovery time afterward. Even a few hours of solitude can help you recharge and restore your energy. Don't feel guilty about needing time to unwind after social interactions.

3. Quality Over Quantity:
Focus on meaningful, quality interactions rather than trying to maintain a high quantity of social engagements. Spend time with people who truly nourish you and support your emotional well-being, rather than trying to keep up with every invitation or demand.

4. Be Honest About Your Needs:
If you're invited to something but feel like you're already reaching your socializing limit, it's okay to say no. You don't have to attend every event or meeting. Simply say, "I'd love to join, but I need some time to recharge today."

5. Use Technology to Stay Connected (on Your Terms):
If socializing in person is draining, stay connected virtually with loved ones in a way that feels manageable. A quick phone call, text, or video chat

can often provide meaningful connection without overwhelming you.

The Takeaway

Emotional boundaries are just as important as physical ones when it comes to avoiding burnout. Protecting yourself from draining relationships, letting go of people-pleasing, and knowing your Minimum Effective Dose for socializing can help you preserve your energy. By practicing these strategies, you can maintain your emotional well-being, avoid burnout, and focus on relationships that nourish and support you. Prioritizing your emotional health is not selfish—it's essential for living a balanced and thriving life.

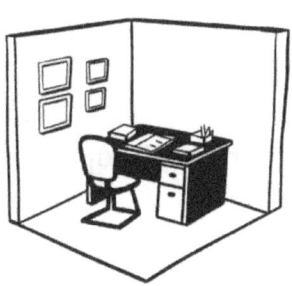

Hello!

Before you begin your Chapter 4 challenge, it would really mean a lot to me if you spent a few minutes and left a book review.

I am a self-published author and one of the best ways for me to get feedback is from you so that I can continue to write and publish books that help improve our lives.

Amazon US:

Thank you once again and I hope you enjoy the rest of the book.

With warmest wishes and sending love your way,

Andrea Sinclair

Your Chapter 4 Challenge: Emotional Boundaries Reset

In this challenge, you will practice setting emotional boundaries in your personal and professional relationships, and begin prioritizing yourself without guilt. These steps will help you protect your emotional energy, reduce people-pleasing behaviors, and manage draining relationships so that you can focus on what truly nourishes you.

Step 1: Identify Your Energy Vampires

Take a moment to reflect on the people in your life who consistently drain your energy. This could be a colleague, friend, or family member. Write down three individuals who tend to leave you feeling emotionally exhausted after spending time with them. For each person, note what specific behaviors or patterns contribute to this drain.

Action:

- Set a boundary with one of these individuals. Use one of the scripts provided earlier to communicate your limits. For example, if someone is constantly venting to you, say, "I understand you're going through a tough time, but I'm feeling overwhelmed right now. Let's talk about it at a time when I can fully listen."

Step 2: Practice the 24-Hour Rule (No Overcommitting)

Many of us say "yes" to things before fully thinking about how it will impact our time and energy. Today, try the 24-Hour Rule: if someone asks you for a commitment or favors, tell them, "Let me check my schedule and get back to you tomorrow." This will give you the space to consider whether it's something that aligns with your priorities and energy levels.

Action:

- The next time someone asks you for something you feel uncertain about committing to, use this phrase and then take the time to evaluate your needs.
- Reflect on how it feels to say "no" or delay your response. Were you surprised by the amount of guilt you felt? Challenge yourself to notice those feelings and remind yourself that your needs matter.

Step 3: Practice the "Minimum Effective Dose" in Socializing

Socializing can either recharge you or drain you, so this week, experiment with your Minimum Effective Dose for social interaction. Pay attention to how much socializing is enough for you. Do you feel energized or exhausted after meeting up with friends or attending events? Start to identify patterns in how much socializing you can handle before you feel depleted.

Action:

- This week, limit your socializing to what feels right for you. Choose one event or social gathering that you

would normally attend, and either cancel or leave early to honor your energy limits.
- If you need to, have a prepared response ready, like: "I'm so glad we could spend time together, but I need to leave to recharge. Let's catch up again soon." This can help you practice balancing social time with personal space without guilt.

Step 4: End the Day with a Boundaries Reset

Set a clear boundary at the end of each workday and social interaction. This will be your mental separation from work and other obligations. It's essential to give yourself a true break in order to recharge emotionally.

Action:

- Decide on a ritual for your "end of day" transition. This could be something as simple as closing your laptop and going for a walk, or taking a few moments to journal.
- When the workday or social activity ends, do your ritual and fully disconnect for the rest of the evening, whether that means taking a break from email or turning off your phone. Observe how this boundary affects your emotional well-being and productivity the next day.

Your Reflection:

At the end of the week, take a moment to reflect on your experience:

- How did setting emotional boundaries affect your energy levels?
- What emotions did you feel when you said "no" or practiced the 24-Hour Rule?
- Did you notice a change in how you approached socializing and interactions with others?
- How do you feel about the time you created for yourself?

These steps will help you start taking control of your emotional boundaries and begin feeling more balanced in your personal and professional life. Remember, the goal is not perfection, but progress. With each small step, you'll begin to reclaim your energy and reduce burnout from emotional drain.

Chapter 5

Mental Resilience—Rewiring Your Mind to Handle Stress Better

"Burnout isn't just about doing too much—it's about how you handle what life throws at you. The strongest people don't avoid stress, they manage it differently."

5.1 The Burnout-Proof Mindset—How Resilient People Think

In the battle against burnout, mindset can be the difference between thriving and surviving. Resilience—the ability to bounce back from challenges and maintain your well-being under stress—isn't just about having a strong constitution or a tough attitude. It's about cultivating the right mental framework. In this section, we'll dive into how resilient people think and the mental shifts you can make to protect yourself from burnout.

Let's explore the key elements that make up a burnout-proof mindset: understanding the power of mindset itself, navigating cognitive overload, and learning how to detach from stress so you can gain control over your thoughts.

The Growth vs. Fixed Mindset: Why Your Response to Stress Matters More Than Stress Itself

The way we view challenges can either empower or trap us. According to psychologist Carol Dweck, there are two fundamental types of mindsets: growth and fixed. How you respond to stress is largely shaped by which mindset you adopt.

1. Fixed Mindset:
    People with a fixed mindset believe that their abilities, intelligence, and skills are set in stone. They view challenges as threats and failures as evidence of their limitations. When stress arises, they might feel overwhelmed or defeated because they believe they can't handle it.

2. Growth Mindset:
    In contrast, those with a growth mindset believe that they can develop their abilities over time. They see challenges as opportunities to learn and grow, and they embrace the discomfort that comes with change and progress. When stress hits, they view it as a temporary hurdle they can overcome with effort, adaptability, and perseverance.

Action:

- Take a moment to reflect on how you typically respond to stress. Do you feel defeated when faced

with a challenge, or do you see it as an opportunity to learn and adapt?
- Moving forward, when a stressful situation arises, consciously choose to adopt a growth mindset. Tell yourself, "This is hard, but it's an opportunity to grow. I can figure this out and come out stronger."

Cognitive Load vs. Physical Load: Understanding Mental Fatigue and How to Fix It

Many people assume that physical exhaustion is the primary cause of burnout. While physical fatigue is important, mental fatigue—the strain from cognitive overload—often plays a bigger role in burnout. Your mind, like your body, can only handle so much before it needs a break.

Cognitive load refers to the mental effort required to perform tasks. It's the strain on your brain from making decisions, processing information, and managing multiple thoughts at once. Over time, high cognitive load can lead to mental fatigue, which reduces your ability to think clearly, make decisions, and stay productive.

1. Recognize Mental Overload:
   Mental fatigue often manifests as difficulty concentrating, forgetfulness, irritability, and a feeling of being mentally "stuck." If you've ever felt like you're spinning your wheels, unable to think clearly even though you've been working hard, it's likely due to cognitive overload.

2. Reducing Cognitive Load:

   - Simplify Decisions: Create routines for tasks that don't require a lot of thought. This reduces the number of decisions you need to make throughout the day.
   - Take Mental Breaks: Schedule regular pauses in your day to clear your mind. Even a 5-minute walk or a few minutes of deep breathing can help reset your brain and restore your focus.
   - Batch Similar Tasks: Rather than switching between different types of tasks, group similar ones together. This minimizes the mental energy required to transition between tasks.

Action:

- For the next 3 days, track your mental fatigue. At the end of each day, ask yourself:
    - "Did I feel mentally drained today?"
    - "Was I jumping between tasks too often?"
    - "Could I have simplified any decisions or tasks?"
    - Commit to one change that will reduce your cognitive load, whether it's simplifying your schedule or incorporating more breaks.

How to Detach from Stressful Thoughts: Proven Techniques to Stop Overanalyzing Everything

Stress often begins in the mind. When you're overwhelmed, it's easy to become trapped in a spiral of overthinking—constantly analyzing, worrying, and replaying scenarios in your head. This can heighten feelings of stress, anxiety, and burnout. The key to breaking this cycle is learning how to detach from those stress-driven thoughts.

Here are some effective techniques for detaching from stressful thinking patterns:

1. Mindfulness and Present-Moment Awareness: Mindfulness is the practice of bringing your attention to the present moment. By focusing on your breath, bodily sensations, or the world around you, you can break free from the constant stream of stress-driven thoughts. This helps you become more grounded and centered, reducing the impact of stress.

2. Cognitive Behavioral Techniques (CBT): Cognitive Behavioral Therapy teaches us to challenge irrational or unproductive thoughts. When you catch yourself overanalyzing or catastrophizing, pause and ask yourself, "What evidence do I have for this thought? Is this helpful? What is the worst-case scenario, and how likely is it to happen?" This can help you reframe your thinking.

3. The "Stop" Technique:
When you notice yourself spiraling into overthinking, practice saying "Stop" out loud (or in your head). Then redirect your attention to something more constructive or calming, like a task, a conversation, or

simply breathing deeply. This interruption prevents you from going deeper into stress.

4. Thought Journaling:
   Writing down your thoughts helps to externalize them, putting them on paper so you can better analyze them. This can provide clarity and perspective, making it easier to let go of thoughts that are adding to your stress.

Action:

- Choose one technique (mindfulness, CBT, the "Stop" technique, or thought journaling) and practice it every day for the next week.
- Pay attention to how your ability to detach from stressful thoughts improves, and how this shift impacts your stress levels and your ability to stay grounded.

The Takeaway

Building a burnout-proof mindset is about understanding how your thoughts influence your response to stress. By shifting from a fixed mindset to a growth mindset, managing cognitive load, and practicing techniques to detach from stressful thinking, you can build resilience and prevent burnout. It's not the stress itself that causes burnout—it's how you handle it. With the right mindset and tools, you can face challenges with greater ease, bounce back from setbacks, and protect your mental health from the exhausting cycle of overthinking.

5.2 The Power of Emotional Regulation—How to Stay Calm Under Pressure

In moments of high stress, how you manage your emotions can make or break your ability to function effectively. Emotional regulation—the ability to control and adjust your emotional state—is key to staying calm under pressure and preventing burnout. It's not about suppressing your emotions, but rather learning to respond to them in a way that helps you stay balanced, focused, and clear-headed.

In this section, we'll explore why typical strategies, like deep breathing alone, aren't always enough and dive into neuroscience-backed techniques that are more effective in calming your nervous system. We'll also cover quick methods for resetting during stressful moments and how to manage anxiety when you're in high-pressure situations.

Why Deep Breathing Alone Doesn't Work (And What Does)

While deep breathing is often recommended for stress relief, it's not always the miracle solution many believe it to be—

especially when you're dealing with intense emotions. Deep breathing can help, but it's not the only mechanism your body needs to truly calm down, especially when you're in fight-or-flight mode.

1. The Problem with Shallow Breathing:
   When you're stressed, your body naturally shifts to shallow, rapid breathing, which can perpetuate the stress response. Deep breathing can help reverse this, but to truly address the root cause of your stress, you need more than just deep breaths.

2. Why It's Not Enough:
   Deep breathing alone doesn't fully address the neurochemistry of stress. When you're under pressure, your body releases stress hormones like cortisol and adrenaline, which prepare you to fight or flee. But this can lead to tension, anxiety, and difficulty thinking clearly. To calm your nervous system effectively, you need techniques that activate the parasympathetic nervous system, the body's natural "rest and digest" mode.

3. What Works:
   - Grounding Techniques: These focus on reconnecting you with the present moment by using your senses. A quick grounding exercise could involve feeling the texture of an object in your hand or noticing the temperature around you.

- Movement and Posture: Research shows that shifting your posture can help calm your body. Standing up straight, taking a slow walk, or doing gentle stretching can be more effective at relieving stress than simply sitting and breathing.
  - Progressive Muscle Relaxation (PMR): This technique involves tensing and relaxing muscle groups to release physical tension and trigger the relaxation response. It helps break the cycle of stress by physically lowering your body's tension levels.

Action:

- Today, experiment with Progressive Muscle Relaxation for 5 minutes. Start by tensing your feet for a few seconds, then release. Slowly work your way up through your body (legs, abdomen, arms, shoulders, and face) and feel the tension melt away with each release.

The 10-Second Reset: A Fast, Simple Way to Interrupt Stress Spirals

When you're caught in a stress spiral, it feels nearly impossible to regain control. But there's a quick and effective technique that can interrupt the cycle of stress and bring you back to a place of calm in just 10 seconds.

The 10-Second Reset is a simple but powerful technique that allows you to stop the rapid stream of anxious thoughts or physiological reactions. Here's how it works:

1. **Pause and Breathe:**
   In the midst of a stressful moment, immediately take a deep, intentional breath in. Hold it for a moment, then release it slowly. The act of breathing out slowly helps signal your body to shift out of the fight-or-flight response.

2. **Shift Your Focus:**
   In that same 10 seconds, redirect your attention to something grounding. This could be the feel of your feet on the ground, the sensation of your hands resting on a surface, or simply noticing your surroundings. This helps break the cycle of spiraling thoughts.

3. **Quick Affirmation:**
   End the reset with a short, positive affirmation. Something like, "I'm in control," or "This moment is temporary, and I can handle it." This reinforces your ability to manage the situation and primes your brain for calm.

Action:

- The next time you feel stress rising, try the 10-Second Reset:
    - Breathe in deeply for 4 seconds.

- Exhale slowly for 6 seconds.
- Reconnect with the present moment using your senses and reaffirm your control over the situation.

• Practice this once today—and notice how it helps you gain control over a stressful moment.

How to Manage Anxiety in High-Stress Situations: Practical Tools for Instant Relief

Anxiety often comes with intense physical sensations, such as rapid heartbeats, shallow breathing, or a racing mind. In high-stress situations—whether it's a presentation, difficult conversation, or looming deadline—having tools on hand to manage anxiety is essential.

Here are some practical techniques to help you regain control and calm your nerves:

1. Box Breathing:
    This is a variation of deep breathing that's especially effective for anxiety. It involves inhaling for 4 seconds, holding the breath for 4 seconds, exhaling for 4 seconds, and holding for 4 seconds before starting again. This method helps regulate your breath, calm your nervous system, and refocus your mind.

2. Visualization:
    Visualization is a powerful tool to reduce anxiety. Close your eyes and imagine yourself in a peaceful, relaxing place—whether it's a beach, forest, or

somewhere else that brings you calm. Engage all of your senses: imagine the smell of the air, the sounds around you, the colors you see, and the sensations of touch. This mental escape can reduce the immediate anxiety and help you gain a sense of control.

3. The 5-4-3-2-1 Grounding Exercise: This technique brings you into the present moment by using your senses. It's especially useful when anxiety makes you feel disconnected from reality. To do this:

    - 5: Name five things you can see around you.
    - 4: Name four things you can touch or feel.
    - 3: Name three things you can hear.
    - 2: Name two things you can smell.
    - 1: Name one thing you can taste. This exercise helps pull you out of your anxious thoughts and brings your mind back to reality.

Action:

- Choose one of the above tools and use it next time you experience anxiety or find yourself in a high-stress situation. Practice it daily for the next week to see how it impacts your anxiety levels.

The Takeaway

Emotional regulation is about having the tools to stay calm under pressure and effectively manage stress. Techniques like deep breathing, grounding, and visualization can help you regain your balance and protect your mental well-being. By practicing these methods, you'll be able to interrupt stress spirals, manage anxiety in real-time, and calm your nervous system when you need it most. With consistent practice, emotional regulation will become second nature, enabling you to maintain your energy and resilience—even in the most challenging moments.

Arianna's Moment of Calm:

Arianna had just returned from a high-stakes meeting at work where tensions were running high. She was leading a project that could potentially secure a major client for her company, but things weren't going as smoothly as she had hoped. The client had raised concerns, her team was scrambling to come up with answers, and her boss was looking to her for reassurance.

As the meeting wrapped up, Arianna felt her heart rate spike. She had the familiar rush of anxiety—the feeling of not being able to breathe deeply, the tightness in her chest, and the swirl of negative thoughts racing in her mind. The pressure of the situation was mounting, and she could feel herself on the brink of a stress spiral.

But then, Arianna remembered the 10-Second Reset.

She stepped into the hallway, took a deep breath in for 4 seconds, held it for a beat, and then exhaled slowly for 6 seconds. Immediately, she noticed her body begin to shift. The tension in her shoulders eased. She felt her heartbeat slow down. She then shifted her attention to the sounds of the office around her—the hum of the air conditioner, the faint murmur of colleagues in the next room.

Arianna gave herself a moment to let go of the urgency and reminded herself, "I'm in control. I've handled tough situations before, and I can handle this one too."

With that, she felt a shift in her thinking. She no longer felt overwhelmed by the meeting or the high expectations. The reset had cleared her mind, helping her shift from anxious thinking to a more grounded and clear state.

When she re-entered the office, she was able to approach the problem with a level head. She quickly scheduled a follow-up meeting with her team, reassured her boss with a plan of action, and felt empowered to take the next steps—confidently and without letting the stress overwhelm her.

Arianna's ability to reset in that critical moment not only helped her regain composure but also shifted her mindset from reactive to proactive. She realized that even in the most high-pressure situations, emotional regulation could give her the space she needed to handle the stress, rather than letting the stress handle her.

This story illustrates how taking a brief moment to practice a quick emotional regulation technique like the 10-Second Reset can create a shift in mindset and calm even the most stressful moments.

5.3 Mental Detox—Eliminating Thought Patterns That Drain You

Our minds are powerful, but they can also be our biggest source of stress and burnout. Thoughts, especially the unhelpful ones, have a tendency to cycle—replaying worst-case scenarios, striving for perfection, or endlessly seeking control over things we can't change. In this section, we'll explore how to detoxify your mind by breaking free from thought patterns that drain your energy and keep you stuck in a loop of stress and overwhelm.

By learning how to break the overthinking habit, stop the cycle of perfectionism, and embrace the art of letting go, you'll create mental space for more peace and productivity. Let's dive in and start clearing the mental clutter that holds you back from truly thriving.

Breaking the Overthinking Habit: How to Stop Replaying Worst-Case Scenarios

Overthinking is a mental trap that so many of us fall into, especially when we're stressed. The more we think, the more we spin out, imagining the worst possible outcomes and getting lost in an endless loop of "what ifs." This constant rumination can heighten anxiety, waste mental energy, and keep us stuck in the stress cycle.

1. The Cycle of Overthinking:
    Overthinking often happens when we feel uncertain or out of control. We try to solve problems by mentally rehearsing every possible scenario, but instead of finding solutions, we end up amplifying our stress. It's a mental hamster wheel, where the harder we try to

find answers, the more we feel trapped in anxiety.

2. The Secret to Breaking the Cycle:

    - Set Time Limits for Thinking: One of the most effective ways to combat overthinking is to set a thinking limit. When a stressful thought arises, allow yourself 10 minutes to fully explore the issue. After that, you have to move on. This creates a boundary for your mind and helps break the habit of mental overdrive.
    - Shift to Action: Overthinking can only be stopped by doing something—even if it's just a small step. Action creates momentum and breaks the cycle of analysis paralysis.
    - Distraction and Refocus: When your mind starts to spiral into overthinking, consciously distract yourself by doing something else. Watch a show, take a walk, or engage in a creative activity. When you return to the issue, you'll have a refreshed perspective.

Action:

- The next time you catch yourself overthinking, set a 10-minute timer to focus on the problem. After that, give yourself permission to let it go or take action. Notice how this boundary helps you break free from the cycle of rumination.

The Perfectionist's Dilemma: How to Stop Burnout Caused by Unrealistic Standards

Perfectionism is a silent saboteur of our well-being. It's the driving force behind the pressure we place on ourselves to meet impossibly high standards, often leading to feelings of inadequacy, burnout, and exhaustion. Perfectionists tend to believe that their worth is tied to their achievements and how flawless their work is. This belief creates constant stress and a never-ending desire to control every detail.

1. Why Perfectionism is Exhausting: Perfectionism drives you to strive for an impossible ideal, leaving you never satisfied with your performance. This leads to burnout because you are continually running at full speed without feeling any relief. Even when you do well, it's never enough. You're always pushing to do more, be better, and avoid mistakes.

2. How to Overcome Perfectionism:

    - Shift to "Good Enough" Thinking: Embrace the concept of "good enough" instead of aiming for perfection. The goal is to make progress, not to achieve flawlessness. Ask yourself: "Is this the best I can do right now?" If it is, then allow yourself to move forward without obsessing over the details.
    - Set Realistic Expectations: Recognize that human limitations are part of the equation. You can aim high without demanding the impossible. Setting more realistic goals can

help prevent burnout and lead to healthier progress.
- Celebrate Effort Over Results: Instead of focusing solely on outcomes, shift your focus to effort. Acknowledge and celebrate the energy, time, and intention you put into your work, regardless of whether it's perfect.

Action:

- Identify one area of your life where perfectionism is draining you—whether at work, home, or in your personal relationships. Set a "good enough" goal for the next task and focus on completing it without obsessing over every detail. Notice how the pressure lifts once you release the need for perfection.

The Science of Letting Go: Why Learning to Release Control Reduces Stress

Many of us carry an invisible burden: the need to control everything. Whether it's the outcome of a project, how others behave, or even our own emotions, we often feel an overwhelming desire to micromanage the details of our lives. This desire to control, however, is a major contributor to stress and burnout.

The science of letting go tells us that releasing control can have profound effects on reducing anxiety and stress. When we let go of the need to control every aspect of our lives, we open ourselves to greater peace, creativity, and resilience.

1. Control vs. Adaptability:
   Research shows that when we focus on controlling uncontrollable factors, we increase stress hormones like cortisol and adrenaline. In contrast, when we adopt a mindset of adaptability, we're more able to roll with the punches and respond to challenges with ease. The more we try to control, the more anxious we become, whereas accepting uncertainty allows us to manage stress better.

2. How to Let Go of Control:

   - Focus on What You Can Control: The first step in letting go of control is identifying what's actually within your control. You can control your response, your choices, and your effort—but not the outcome or other people's actions. By focusing on your own actions, you can ease the pressure you place on yourself.
   - Practice Acceptance: Embrace the uncertainty of life. Instead of trying to micromanage every situation, accept that things will not always go according to plan. You don't need to control every detail; you just need to respond well to whatever comes your way.
   - Mindfulness and Surrender: Mindfulness practices help you stay present and surrender the need for control. When you observe your thoughts without judgment, you can see the control patterns and gently let them go. Practice surrendering to the flow of life,

recognizing that not everything needs to be tightly held onto.

Action:

- Identify one situation in your life where you are trying to control outcomes. Practice letting go of that control for one week—allow the process to unfold without intervening. Take note of how it feels to release control and notice any changes in your stress levels.

The Takeaway

Mental detox is about creating a clearer, more focused mind by releasing unhelpful thought patterns. Whether you're dealing with overthinking, perfectionism, or the need to control, these mental habits can keep you trapped in a cycle of stress and burnout. By adopting healthier thought patterns—setting boundaries around your thinking, embracing progress over perfection, and practicing the art of letting go—you can free up mental space for creativity, calm, and clarity. It's time to start clearing the clutter in your mind and give yourself the mental room to thrive.

Your Chapter 5 Challenge: The Mental Detox Week

This week, you're going to detox your mind by tackling three key areas: overthinking, perfectionism, and the need for control. These thought patterns can drain your energy and keep you stuck, but with intentional practice, you'll start to break free and regain mental clarity.

Your 3-Step Challenge:

1. **Break the Overthinking Cycle:**
   The next time you catch yourself replaying worst-case scenarios, set a 10-minute timer to think through the issue. After that, shift focus to something else—whether it's taking a walk, diving into a task, or engaging in something creative. This will give you mental space and prevent endless rumination.

2. **Challenge Perfectionism:**
   Identify one task (either at work or in your personal life) that you tend to perfect. Set a "good enough" goal for that task and allow yourself to move on after completion. Celebrate the effort you put in, instead of focusing solely on the outcome.

3. **Let Go of Control:**
   This week, find one area of your life where you're trying to control outcomes (e.g., a work project or a situation with a friend). Practice releasing control—let things unfold naturally without intervening.

Notice how it feels to surrender and observe how your stress levels change.

Daily Reflection:

At the end of each day, take a few minutes to reflect on what worked and how it felt to practice these mental detox techniques. Write down any shifts you noticed in your stress, mental clarity, and overall sense of calm.

By completing this Mental Detox Week, you'll begin to shift your thinking, reduce stress, and create a more balanced, resilient mindset. Ready to detox your mind? Let's get started!

A Free Thank You Gift

As a token of my appreciation and a way of saying thanks for your purchase, I'm offering the short book **Sleep Your Way to Balance: Nighttime Rituals to Recharge Your Body and Mind** for FREE to my readers.

To get instant access scan the QR code or just go to:

https://andreasinclairbooks.com/free-gift

Inside the book, you will discover:

- Nighttime Rituals to Recharge
- Science-backed Tips and Tricks
- 30 Minute Wind Down Formula

If you want to improve your sleep and feel better, make sure to grab the free book!

Chapter 6

Purpose and Meaning—How to Reignite Motivation and Joy

"Burnout isn't just physical exhaustion—it's emotional exhaustion. When life feels meaningless, no amount of rest will fix it. Let's bring the spark back."

6.1 The Burnout-Purpose Connection—Why We Burn Out When We Lose Meaning

It's no secret that burnout often feels like more than just physical exhaustion—it's the kind of deep, soul-draining fatigue that leaves you wondering, Is this it? You can work long hours, push through stress, and juggle countless tasks, but if what you're doing lacks meaning or purpose, it's easy to feel like you're running on empty.

In this section, we'll explore the connection between purpose and burnout—why a lack of purpose can make burnout even worse, how to rediscover the passion that fuels you, and why joy and fulfillment come from more than just relaxation.

The Hedonic vs. Eudaimonic Happiness Debate: Why Joy Comes from More Than Just Relaxation

Hedonic happiness is the type of joy that comes from pleasure, comfort, and relaxation—the things that make you feel good in the moment. We often seek this kind of happiness in things like vacations, good food, or simply chilling out. While this kind of happiness isn't bad, it has a short shelf life. It feels great in the moment but doesn't always leave us feeling deeply fulfilled.

On the other hand, eudaimonic happiness is rooted in a sense of purpose, personal growth, and contributing to something greater than oneself. This type of happiness comes from pursuing things that align with our values, helping others, or mastering a skill. Unlike hedonic pleasure, which fades quickly, eudaimonic happiness has lasting power. It's the kind of fulfillment that gives you energy rather than draining it.

1. The Hedonic Trap of Burnout: When you're burnt out, it's easy to think that all you need is more rest or more "me time." While relaxation is essential, it doesn't always address the deeper cause of your exhaustion—the lack of meaning in your daily activities. If your life is full of hedonic pursuits but lacks a sense of purpose, you'll likely still feel unfulfilled, no matter how much downtime you have.

2. Eudaimonic Joy and Burnout Recovery: To truly recover from burnout, it's important to incorporate eudaimonic elements back into your

life—things that give you a sense of purpose, growth, and contribution. When you reconnect with activities that align with your core values, you'll feel more energized and motivated, and the cycle of burnout can start to reverse.

The "Purpose Deficit" of Burnout: How Losing Sight of Why You Work Makes Exhaustion Worse

Purpose is what drives us—it's the reason we get up in the morning and face the challenges ahead. But when you're burnt out, it's easy to forget why you do what you do. Your work may feel like an endless to-do list, rather than a meaningful contribution to your goals or the world around you.

1. Why Purpose Deficit Leads to Burnout: A lack of purpose at work or in life creates a void—a feeling of being disconnected from the things that truly matter. The more disconnected you feel from your work, the more exhaustion sets in. If you can't see how your efforts are contributing to a bigger picture, it's easy to feel depleted and frustrated.

2. The Spiral of Exhaustion:
When you lose sight of your purpose, the work becomes just a grind—and the grind will always lead to burnout. Without purpose, the energy you spend feels wasted, and the joy you once found in your work evaporates. It's a vicious cycle: the more disconnected you feel from your purpose, the more drained you

become, until you reach a point where you can't summon the energy to care anymore.

How to Reconnect with What Actually Fulfills You: Rediscovering Passion Without Needing a Major Life Overhaul

It's not necessary to make a massive life change to rediscover your passion and reconnect with purpose. In fact, small shifts and intentional reflection can help you start moving toward greater fulfillment without completely overhauling your life. The key is to start with small, manageable steps.

1. Reflect on Your Values:
   Take a moment to think about what truly matters to you. What are the things that make you feel alive and energized? What values are most important to you? The more you identify these values, the clearer your sense of purpose will become. Purpose isn't something that's fixed or external—it's an evolving process of aligning what you do with what truly matters to you.

2. Incorporate Meaning into Your Daily Life:
   You don't need to quit your job or radically change your career to reconnect with purpose. Start by asking yourself, How can I add more meaning to my current role? Whether it's helping a colleague, creating something impactful, or focusing on aspects of your work that align with your values, small changes can

reignite your sense of purpose.

3. Pursue Passion Projects:
   Beyond work, think about activities or hobbies that you're passionate about. Pursuing passion projects, even if they're small and outside of your day-to-day responsibilities, can reignite a sense of fulfillment. Whether it's volunteering, learning a new skill, or working on a personal project, these activities will help fill the "purpose gap" that burnout creates.

The Takeaway

When you're burnt out, the lack of purpose is often at the heart of your exhaustion. While relaxation and self-care are vital for recovery, the deeper cause of burnout lies in a disconnect from the meaning behind your work and life. Reconnecting with purpose—whether by identifying your core values, finding meaningful tasks within your current life, or pursuing passion projects outside of work—can help you rediscover the energy and motivation you've been missing. Purpose is the antidote to burnout, and it doesn't require a drastic life overhaul. You can start small and build from there, and in doing so, you'll begin to feel more fulfilled, energized, and aligned with what truly matters.

Example: Sarah's Journey to Rediscovering Purpose

Sarah had been working in marketing for over 12 years, but lately, everything felt like a grind. She was tired all the time, no matter how many hours she spent resting on the weekends. She'd wake up feeling drained and unmotivated, staring at her to-do list, dreading the day ahead. Her job, which used to excite her, now felt like an endless cycle of emails, meetings, and reports.

One morning, Sarah realized that part of the problem wasn't her workload—it was that she had lost sight of why she was doing it all in the first place. She had once felt driven by the creative aspects of her job, but as the years passed, the focus had shifted to endless tasks and meeting deadlines. She felt disconnected from the bigger picture, from the purpose that had once fueled her.

Determined to get back on track, Sarah took a step back and asked herself, What really matters to me? After reflecting on her values, she realized that creativity, helping others, and making an impact were at the core of what she wanted to do. The problem wasn't the work itself, but how she had lost the connection between her daily tasks and her larger values.

She began by looking for ways to add more meaning to her current role. In team meetings, she started suggesting more creative approaches to projects and pushed for opportunities to collaborate with her colleagues on initiatives that had a deeper purpose. She realized that by focusing on tasks that allowed her to be more creative and innovative, she reignited her sense of fulfillment.

At the same time, Sarah made space for passion projects outside of work. She had always loved photography, so she decided to take an online course and dedicate weekends to practicing. This simple change filled her with a new sense of passion, and she began to feel more energized throughout the week. Her work didn't feel as draining anymore because she had rediscovered the joy and creativity that had originally drawn her to marketing.

Over time, Sarah found that she no longer needed to make a major life overhaul to reconnect with purpose. By identifying her core values, finding meaning in her current job, and pursuing passions outside of work, she created a more balanced, fulfilling life. The burnout that had once felt overwhelming started to fade, replaced by a renewed sense of purpose and excitement.

Sarah's story illustrates that burnout often arises when we lose sight of the deeper meaning behind what we do. By reconnecting with our core values and seeking out activities that align with our sense of purpose—whether in our work or personal lives—we can find our way back to energy, joy, and fulfillment without needing a complete life overhaul.

6.2 Finding Fulfillment in the Everyday—How to Make Any Job More Meaningful

We often think that fulfillment comes only from big changes—like a new career, a fresh start, or a major life overhaul. But what if I told you that you don't need to leave your job or upend your life to find meaning and purpose? The truth is, meaning can be found right where you are, in the everyday moments of your work. The key is understanding how to craft your job to align with what truly excites and fulfills you.

In this section, we'll explore three powerful ways to rediscover fulfillment in your daily work: job crafting, micro-wins, and the Ikigai method. With these tools, you can bring passion, purpose, and energy back to any job—whether you're in a role you love or one that feels like it's draining you.

Job Crafting: How Small Tweaks in Your Work Can Bring Back Passion

Job crafting is a concept that allows you to reshape your current role to better align with your strengths, passions, and values. Instead of waiting for your job to suddenly become more fulfilling or hoping for a promotion to find purpose, you can take action to craft your job in small, intentional ways.

1. Find What You Love:
   The first step is to identify the parts of your job that bring you joy. Is it working with certain colleagues? Problem-solving in a particular area? Or maybe the creative side of what you do? Whatever it is, make a list of the aspects that energize you and bring you the most satisfaction.

2. Reframe or Add Tasks:
   Once you've identified what you enjoy, think about how you can add more of those elements to your day-to-day work. Maybe you can take on new projects that align with your strengths or find creative ways to

integrate your passions into your current responsibilities. It could be as simple as offering to lead a brainstorming session or adjusting your role to focus more on a specific aspect of your work.

3. **Delegate or Minimize Tasks You Don't Enjoy:** Equally important is identifying the aspects of your job that drain you or feel disconnected from your values. While you may not be able to eliminate them completely, consider if there are tasks you can delegate or minimize. By shifting the balance toward the aspects of your work you enjoy, you can reinvigorate your sense of purpose.

Micro-Wins: The Science Behind Celebrating Small Progress to Feel Re-Energized

In the hustle of daily work, it's easy to feel like you're not making progress—especially when tasks feel overwhelming or endless. But the truth is, small wins are powerful for maintaining energy and motivation. The science behind micro-wins shows that celebrating small achievements can trigger the release of dopamine, the brain's reward chemical, which helps you feel re-energized and motivated to keep going.

1. **Break Down Big Tasks:**
Rather than focusing on the larger, daunting task at hand, break it into smaller, more manageable steps. Completing a small portion of the task and acknowledging your success will create a sense of

momentum and accomplishment.

2. Celebrate Progress, Not Perfection:
   Shift your focus from perfection to progress. When you recognize and celebrate even the smallest steps forward—like finishing an email, solving a problem, or having a successful meeting—you'll build a sense of achievement that can carry you through the day.

3. Track Your Wins:
   Keep a micro-win journal where you jot down even the smallest accomplishments. This practice can help shift your mindset from focusing on what's left to do, to appreciating how much you've already achieved. Over time, you'll notice how this small shift boosts your energy and motivation.

The "Ikigai" Method: How to Align Your Daily Work with What Actually Excites You

Ikigai is a Japanese concept that roughly translates to "a reason for being." It's the idea that true fulfillment comes from aligning what you love, what you're good at, what the world needs, and what you can be paid for. By finding your Ikigai, you can align your work with both your passions and your skills in a way that feels deeply meaningful.

1. Discover Your Ikigai:
   Ask yourself these four key questions:

   o What do I love doing?

- What am I good at?
- What does the world need?
- What can I be paid for?

    Your Ikigai lies at the intersection of these four elements. Even if you're not in your dream job, you can still find ways to align these elements within your current role.

2. Integrate Your Ikigai into Your Daily Work:
   If you're already clear on your Ikigai, look for ways to infuse more of it into your daily work. Are there opportunities to add more of what you love? Can you offer solutions that meet the needs of others while leveraging your strengths? Even the smallest adjustments in your daily routine can bring you closer to a fulfilling life.

3. Reevaluate Over Time:
   Remember that your Ikigai can evolve. What excites you today may shift as you grow. Periodically reevaluate these four areas to ensure that your daily work continues to align with what brings you fulfillment.

The Takeaway

Fulfillment doesn't have to come from a major life change or a new job. By practicing job crafting, celebrating micro-wins, and aligning your work with your Ikigai, you can bring meaning and passion to your daily routine. It's all about finding ways to make your current role fit your strengths and passions, no matter where you are in your career. The key is to take small, intentional steps that connect you to what truly excites you—and with time, you'll find that your work becomes a source of energy and fulfillment instead of a drain.

6.3 Aligning Your Life with Your Values—The Key to Long-Term Balance

In a world that constantly demands more from us—more time, more energy, more attention—it's easy to get swept up in doing things just for the sake of doing them. But true fulfillment and long-term balance don't come from filling every minute with activity or chasing after things that aren't aligned with your core values. Instead, balance comes from embracing the Essentialist mindset—doing less but doing it with more focus, intention, and purpose.

In this section, we'll explore how to align your life with your values in a way that fosters long-term fulfillment and balance. We'll dive into the Essentialist mindset, how to recognize when you're out of alignment with your values, and a simple five-minute daily practice to bring you back to what really matters.

The "Essentialist" Mindset: How Doing Less Can Actually Give You More Fulfillment

The concept of Essentialism is rooted in the idea that by focusing on what truly matters—what adds the most value and meaning to our lives—we can eliminate distractions and find more fulfillment. Instead of doing more to get ahead or prove ourselves, we intentionally choose to focus on fewer, more important things.

1. The Power of "Less":
   Essentialism isn't about laziness or inaction. It's about being deliberate with your time, energy, and efforts. It's recognizing that when you say "yes" to everything, you end up saying "no" to your core values and what truly brings you fulfillment. By doing less, but focusing on the right things, you can experience more joy, impact, and energy in the long run.

2. Creating More Impact by Doing Less:
   When we focus on a few key priorities, we have the time and energy to pour ourselves into them fully. This leads to deeper satisfaction and a higher quality of work and relationships. By aligning with your essential priorities, you can make more of an impact with less effort, leading to greater fulfillment.

3. Letting Go of the "Busy" Trap:
   Our culture celebrates busyness, but the truth is, being busy doesn't always mean you're being productive or fulfilled. The Essentialist mindset encourages you to question the "busy" work and refocus on the things that truly matter. This mindset shift can be transformative in preventing burnout and helping you regain balance in your life.

How to Identify What's Draining You: The Values-Misalignment Checklist

One of the biggest causes of burnout is the feeling of being out of alignment with your values. You may be doing things that look good on paper but don't feel right to you on a deeper level. To reclaim your energy and restore balance, it's crucial to identify where your life might be out of sync with your values.

Here's a Values-Misalignment Checklist to help you identify areas where you might be feeling drained:

1. Does your work feel disconnected from your purpose? Are you going through the motions in your job, but lacking passion for the tasks or the overall mission? If you're not feeling aligned with your work, it can quickly lead to burnout.

2. Are you constantly overcommitting? Are you saying "yes" to things that don't resonate with your values, just to please others or avoid guilt? If your calendar is filled with tasks that don't align with your personal values, you may be draining yourself without realizing it.

3. Are your relationships supportive and fulfilling? Do you feel drained by certain relationships, or are they uplifting and energizing? Relationships that are out of alignment with your values—whether they're demanding or toxic—can contribute to burnout.

4. Do you have time for self-care and relaxation? If you're constantly running on empty and feel guilty for taking time to recharge, it may be a sign that you're misaligned with your need for self-care and balance.

If you find that multiple areas of your life are out of alignment with your values, it's time to take a step back and realign. Identifying these mismatches is the first step in reclaiming balance and restoring your energy.

The 5-Minute Daily Practice for a More Purposeful Life: A Simple Exercise to Realign with What Matters

You don't need to overhaul your life to bring more balance and fulfillment. By integrating small, intentional practices into your day, you can stay aligned with your values and maintain long-term balance. Here's a 5-minute daily practice to help you reconnect with what matters:

1. Set Your Daily Intention (1 minute): Take a moment each morning to identify your intention for the day. What is the one thing that, if you accomplish it, will bring you closer to living your values? Whether it's working on a passion project, setting boundaries, or spending quality time with loved ones, setting an intention keeps you focused on what truly matters.

2. Check In with Your Energy (2 minutes): Throughout your day, pause for 2 minutes to check in with how you're feeling. Are you starting to feel drained or misaligned? This brief pause allows you to assess whether you're still connected to your purpose and values or if you need to adjust your approach.

3. Reflect on Alignment (2 minutes):
At the end of the day, take 2 minutes to reflect on how

well your actions aligned with your core values. Did you prioritize what mattered most to you? Did you stay true to your intention, or did you get swept up in distractions? Use this time to celebrate the small wins and make adjustments for the next day.

By taking just 5 minutes a day to intentionally reconnect with your values, you'll be able to course-correct and maintain balance, without needing to make drastic changes.

The Takeaway

Achieving long-term balance and fulfillment doesn't come from doing more—it comes from aligning your life with what matters most to you. By adopting the Essentialist mindset, identifying areas of misalignment, and practicing a simple daily reflection, you can bring more purpose, energy, and joy into your life. The key is to focus on what truly matters, do less of the things that drain you, and consistently realign with your core values—because balance isn't something you achieve once and for all, it's a continuous practice.

Your Chapter 6 Challenge: Aligning Your Life with Your Values

In this challenge, you'll put the strategies from this chapter into action to find more balance, meaning, and fulfillment in your daily life. By focusing on your values, simplifying your commitments, and aligning your work with what excites you, you'll begin to feel more energized and less overwhelmed. Here's how to get started:

Step 1: The Essentialist Mindset

- Action: Choose one area of your life (work, family, or personal projects) where you feel overextended or misaligned. Ask yourself: "What can I do less of to make room for more of what matters?"
- Example: If work is draining you, think about tasks you can delegate or eliminate. If family commitments are overwhelming, ask yourself where you can set clearer boundaries.

Step 2: Values-Misalignment Checklist

- Action: Review the Values-Misalignment Checklist and reflect on each question. Identify at least one area where you feel out of alignment with your values—whether it's in your work, relationships, or personal habits.
- Example: If you feel disconnected from your work, think about how you could introduce more purpose into your daily tasks. If your relationships feel

draining, decide on one boundary you could set to protect your energy.

Step 3: The 5-Minute Daily Practice

- Action: Commit to a 5-minute daily practice for the next week. Each morning, set an intention for the day based on what aligns with your values, check in with your energy halfway through the day, and reflect on alignment in the evening.
- Example: In the morning, write down your intention (e.g., "Today, I will prioritize deep work that aligns with my core goals"). In the evening, reflect: "Did I stay true to my intention? What drained me? What energized me?"

By completing this challenge, you'll begin to shift your mindset from busyness to purpose, and from overwhelm to intentionality. You'll create space for more fulfillment, leaving you energized and better aligned with what truly matters in your life.

Chapter 7

Sustainable Habits—How to Prevent Burnout from Coming Back

"Burnout recovery isn't just about fixing what's broken—it's about making sure you don't end up here again."

7.1 The Science of Habit Formation—How to Make Changes That Stick

Creating lasting change doesn't come from sheer willpower alone. The truth is, relying on willpower often leads to burnout. Instead, the science of habit formation offers us a much more sustainable way to create new behaviors that stick—and help us avoid burnout in the process. In this section, we'll explore the neuroscience behind habit change, why small, consistent steps are more powerful than major overhauls, and how to stack new habits onto your existing routines for greater success.

Why Willpower Fails (And What Works Instead)

It's a common myth: if you just try harder, you'll get better results. But research shows that willpower has limited capacity—it's like a muscle that gets fatigued after prolonged use. When you rely on willpower to change your habits, it can quickly burn out, leaving you feeling frustrated and stuck. That's why willpower alone isn't the answer.

What works instead is automaticity—the process by which a behavior becomes a routine and requires little to no mental energy. Studies in neuroscience show that habits form in the basal ganglia, the part of the brain responsible for automatic behaviors. The key to lasting change is making small behaviors automatic, so they don't require the constant effort that willpower demands.

The 1% Daily Rule: How Tiny, Daily Improvements Lead to Burnout-Proof Routines

The 1% Daily Rule is one of the most powerful strategies for sustainable habit change. The principle is simple: make tiny improvements every day—just 1%. While 1% may seem small, it compounds over time, leading to dramatic change without the overwhelm of big, sudden efforts.

For example, let's say you want to create a habit of exercising. Instead of committing to a full 30-minute workout every day, start by simply committing to 5 minutes of movement every morning. By focusing on small actions, you create consistency, which builds momentum. Over time, the habit of moving each day becomes automatic, and you can increase the time or intensity as it becomes a natural part of your routine.

This small, consistent approach reduces the likelihood of burnout because you're not overwhelming yourself with drastic changes that require huge amounts of effort upfront.

The Power of Habit Stacking: How to Attach New Habits to Things You're Already Doing

One of the most effective strategies for habit formation is habit stacking. The idea is to attach a new habit to something you're already doing regularly. This takes advantage of the automaticity of your current routines and makes it easier to introduce a new behavior.

For example, if you already drink coffee every morning, you could stack a habit like meditating for 2 minutes right after you finish your coffee. Or, if you brush your teeth every night, you could stack a gratitude practice—simply write down 3 things you're grateful for after brushing.

The key to habit stacking is to make sure the new habit is small, so it feels easy to do and doesn't require significant mental energy. Over time, these small habits will compound and lead to lasting changes that fit seamlessly into your life.

The Takeaway

Creating lasting habits isn't about forcing yourself to stick to rigid routines or relying on willpower. By understanding the neuroscience of habit formation, focusing on 1% daily improvements, and using the power of habit stacking, you can create burnout-proof routines that feel effortless and sustainable. The key is to make small changes that become automatic and integrated into your daily life, so you can sustain progress without overwhelming yourself.

In the next sections, we'll explore how to build on these habits to create lasting change in your life and reduce burnout for good.

7.2 The Energy Budget—How to Balance Work, Rest, and Recovery

In the same way that you manage your financial budget, it's crucial to manage your energy budget. Every day, you have a finite amount of energy to spend—and just like with money, if you spend it all without a plan, you'll quickly find yourself depleted. This section will show you how to track your energy spends, apply the 80/20 rule to cut out unnecessary stress, and create a Recharge Ritual to ensure that you regularly replenish your energy and avoid burnout.

How to Track Your "Energy Spends": Identifying Activities That Drain vs. Restore You

Just as you track your spending to avoid running out of funds, it's important to track how you're spending your energy throughout the day. Every activity you engage in requires a certain amount of energy, and understanding which activities drain you and which ones restore you is key to balancing your energy budget.

1. Identify the Energy Drains:
   Start by tracking your daily activities for a week. Pay attention to moments when you feel drained, exhausted, or stressed. What types of tasks or

interactions lead to these feelings? This could be long meetings, excessive screen time, difficult conversations, or multitasking.

Example: You may realize that back-to-back Zoom meetings leave you feeling exhausted, or that social media scrolling drains your energy by overloading your brain with information.

2. Track the Energy Restores:
Now, pay attention to the activities that make you feel more energized, relaxed, or refreshed. These could include things like taking a walk, journaling, connecting with loved ones, or engaging in hobbies that bring you joy.

Example: You might notice that spending time outdoors or practicing deep breathing helps restore your energy, while a cup of herbal tea or a 10-minute stretch brings you back to life.

By tracking both the energy-draining and energy-restoring activities, you'll have a clearer picture of how your day is shaping your energy levels, which will help you make more intentional choices about how to manage your energy.

The 80/20 Rule for Energy Management: How to Cut Out 80% of Unnecessary Stress

The 80/20 rule, also known as the Pareto Principle, suggests that 80% of your results come from 20% of your efforts.

When applied to energy management, this means that 80% of your energy drains come from just 20% of your activities. Similarly, 80% of your energy restores likely comes from 20% of the things you do.

1. Identify the 20% of Activities That Drain You the Most:
   After tracking your energy spends, look at the activities that are causing the most significant drain. Are there particular tasks, people, or situations that consistently sap your energy? These are the areas where you can make the biggest impact.

2. Eliminate or Minimize Energy Drains:
   Once you've identified the biggest energy drains, think about how you can reduce or eliminate them. This could mean delegating tasks, saying no to unnecessary commitments, or setting stronger boundaries around certain activities that leave you feeling drained.

3. Focus on the 20% That Restores You:
   Next, look at the activities that give you the most energy and focus on them. If taking a 15-minute walk every afternoon helps recharge you, make sure to prioritize that time. If you feel restored after reading or meditating, incorporate those practices into your daily routine.

By applying the 80/20 rule, you can reduce unnecessary stress and focus more of your energy on the things that truly restore and energize you, allowing you to balance work and recovery more effectively.

How to Create a "Recharge Ritual": The Importance of Scheduled, Guilt-Free Rest

Many people struggle to take rest because they feel guilty or think they should always be doing something productive. But scheduled, guilt-free rest is essential for maintaining energy and avoiding burnout. The key is to create a Recharge Ritual—a dedicated, intentional time each day for rest and rejuvenation.

1. **Set Boundaries Around Rest**: Just like you would schedule a work meeting or a family commitment, schedule time for rest and recovery. Whether it's a 20-minute nap, a daily walk, or a quiet hour of reading, block off this time on your calendar as non-negotiable.

2. **Make Your Recharge Ritual Enjoyable:** Your Recharge Ritual should be something you genuinely look forward to. It's not about forcing yourself to "rest" in ways that feel like a chore. Instead, choose activities that nourish you—whether that's meditating, journaling, soaking in a bath, or even just lying in silence.

3. **Embrace Guilt-Free Rest:** Let go of any guilt associated with rest. Remind yourself that rest is productive—it's an investment in your energy and well-being. When you rest, you allow

your brain and body to recover and perform better when you're back at work or in your day-to-day life.

By incorporating a Recharge Ritual into your routine, you give yourself permission to rest without guilt, helping you balance work and recovery, and ensuring that you're consistently recharging your energy.

The Takeaway

Just as a financial budget helps you manage money, an energy budget helps you balance the demands of work, rest, and recovery. By tracking your energy spends, applying the 80/20 rule to eliminate unnecessary drains, and committing to a Recharge Ritual, you can avoid burnout and maintain long-term vitality. Managing your energy isn't about doing more—it's about doing less of what drains you and more of what restores you, ensuring that you always have the energy you need to thrive.

The Energy Audit and Recharge Ritual

1. Track Your Energy Spends: For the next week, track your daily activities and note when you feel drained or restored. Identify at least one activity that consistently drains you and one activity that consistently recharges you.

2. Apply the 80/20 Rule: Review your energy audit and apply the 80/20 rule. Identify the 20% of activities that drain the most energy and find ways to reduce or

eliminate them. Also, identify the 20% of activities that restore your energy and prioritize them.

3. Create Your Recharge Ritual: Schedule a guilt-free recharge ritual for yourself every day this week. Whether it's a 20-minute nap, a quiet walk, or a relaxing bath, make sure to prioritize this time on your calendar as non-negotiable.

By completing this challenge, you'll have a clearer understanding of how to balance your energy more effectively, create lasting habits of recovery, and prevent burnout for the long term.

7.3 How to Spot Early Signs of Burnout Before It's Too Late

Burnout doesn't usually happen overnight. It's the result of chronic stress, unaddressed exhaustion, and a buildup of daily pressures that accumulate over time. Recognizing the early signs of burnout is crucial for preventing it from escalating into full-blown exhaustion. In this section, we'll explore how to perform a quick self-assessment to gauge your burnout levels, spot the subtle warning signs of "micro-burnout," and develop your Personal Burnout Recovery Plan for sustainable stress management.

The 4-Question Burnout Check-In: A Quick Self-Assessment Tool

To catch burnout before it spirals, it's important to check in with yourself regularly. A quick self-assessment can help you gauge whether you're on the path toward burnout or whether you're already showing signs of it. Use the following 4-Question Burnout Check-In to take a quick pulse on your mental, emotional, and physical health:

1. **How am I feeling physically?**
   Are you feeling consistently tired, no matter how much rest you get? Are you experiencing aches, headaches, or a racing heart when faced with stress? Physical exhaustion is one of the first signs that burnout may be creeping in.

2. **Am I feeling emotionally drained or detached?**
   Do you feel numb, disconnected, or emotionally "checked out" from your work or personal life? Emotional exhaustion is a key indicator that burnout is building.

3. **Do I feel mentally overwhelmed or unfocused?**
   Are you having trouble concentrating? Is decision-making harder than usual? Mental fog and decision fatigue are common early signs of burnout.

4. **Am I losing my sense of purpose or motivation?**
   Are you finding it harder to feel excited about your work or personal goals? Losing motivation or a sense

of purpose is a major sign that burnout may be beginning to take hold.

The "Micro-Burnout" Warning Signs: Subtle Clues That You're Headed Toward Exhaustion

Burnout doesn't always announce itself with dramatic signs. In fact, many people experience micro-burnout—small, subtle signs that build over time before they spiral into more significant exhaustion. Here are some early warning signs to watch for, so you can intervene before burnout takes hold:

- Increased irritability or impatience: You find yourself snapping at others or becoming easily frustrated, even with minor setbacks.

- Constantly feeling "on edge": You can't seem to relax, even during downtime. Your nervous system feels like it's constantly in fight-or-flight mode.

- Reduced enthusiasm for things you usually enjoy: Activities or hobbies that once excited you now feel like chores or burdens. This loss of interest can indicate that your energy reserves are running low.

- Difficulty focusing or making decisions: Your mind feels foggy, and you may procrastinate or feel like you can't make decisions—large or small—without becoming overwhelmed.

- Frequent illnesses or health complaints: A drop in immune function, increased colds, digestive issues, or chronic headaches may signal that your body is fighting stress and fatigue.

If you notice any of these signs, it's essential to take immediate action to prevent full-blown burnout. Even small steps toward self-care can make a significant difference in reversing the early stages of burnout.

Your Personal Burnout Recovery Plan: How to Create a Go-To Strategy for Future Stress

The best way to avoid reaching the point of burnout is to have a preemptive plan in place—a Personal Burnout Recovery Plan. When you begin to notice the warning signs of burnout, you need a strategy to manage your stress and get back on track quickly. Here's how to create your recovery plan:

1. Identify Your Burnout Triggers:
   Reflect on past periods when you've experienced burnout or near-burnout. What were the main triggers? Was it excessive work hours, lack of sleep, or over-commitment? Knowing what causes you to burn out helps you prevent it in the future.

2. Develop Your Action Plan:
   Write down at least three action steps you can take to combat burnout when it's starting to build. These could include things like taking a mental health day, setting clearer boundaries, practicing mindfulness, or

simplifying your schedule. Make sure that these actions are things you can do immediately when burnout is starting to build.

3. Create a Support System:
   Having a network of people to turn to for emotional support is key. This might include a mentor, therapist, friends, or family. Make sure you have someone to talk to when things feel overwhelming.

4. Schedule Regular Check-Ins:
   Make it a habit to check in with yourself weekly or bi-weekly to assess your energy levels and stress. Ask yourself the 4-Question Burnout Check-In. Are you feeling drained? Do you need to adjust your routine or take some time off? Regular check-ins help you catch burnout early before it's too late.

5. Implement Regular Recharge Breaks:
   Incorporate daily or weekly recharge breaks into your schedule—time for reflection, relaxation, and self-care. Whether it's a walk in nature, journaling, or simply doing nothing for 10 minutes, make sure you are regularly recharging.

The Takeaway

Burnout doesn't always give a loud warning before it hits, but by paying attention to the early warning signs and checking in with yourself regularly, you can catch it before it escalates. Use the 4-Question Burnout Check-In to assess your mental, emotional, and physical health. Spot the micro-burnout warning signs that signal trouble ahead, and develop a Personal Burnout Recovery Plan that includes clear actions to prevent and recover from burnout. With this proactive approach, you'll be able to manage stress more effectively, stay ahead of burnout, and maintain lasting energy and vitality.

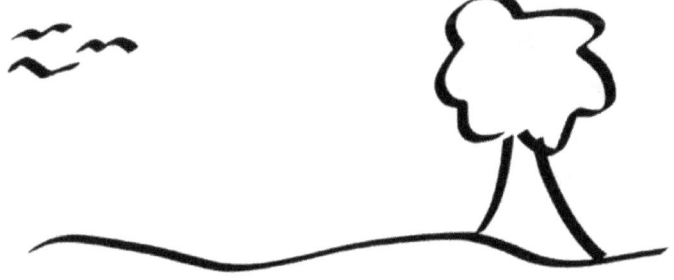

Your Chapter 7 Challenge: Spotting Early Burnout and Creating Your Recovery Plan

1. **Complete the 4-Question Burnout Check-In:** Reflect on how you're feeling in each of the four areas: physical, emotional, mental, and motivation. Do you notice any signs of burnout?

2. **Identify Your Micro-Burnout Warning Signs:** Over the next week, pay attention to any subtle burnout signs (like irritability, foggy thinking, or reduced enthusiasm). Write down what you notice.

3. **Develop Your Personal Burnout Recovery Plan:** Create your action steps to take when burnout shows up (e.g., schedule a mental health day, say no to a commitment, go for a walk). Add a support system you can rely on and set up regular check-ins to monitor your energy levels.

By completing this challenge, you'll be equipped with the tools and strategies to spot burnout early, take immediate action, and keep your energy balanced—no matter what life throws your way.

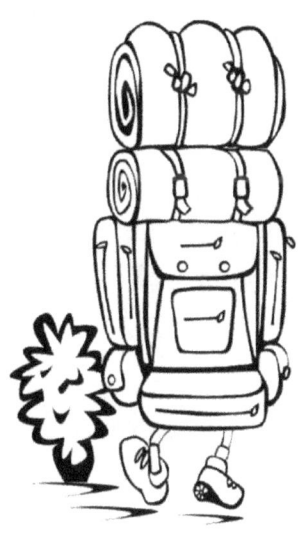

Chapter 8

The 7-Step Burnout Recovery Plan—Your Personalized Blueprint for Balance

"You now have everything you need to break free from burnout. But knowledge alone won't change your life—taking action will."

8.1 Putting It All Together—Your Customizable Burnout Recovery Plan

Creating a personalized burnout recovery plan is your ultimate tool for turning things around and stepping into a life of balance and energy. In this section, we'll walk through the three essential steps to craft your customized recovery strategy that you can revisit whenever burnout starts to creep in. The goal is to not only help you recover from burnout but also to prevent it in the future.

Step 1: Identify Your Burnout Type

The first step in your recovery plan is pinpointing your burnout type. The more specific you can be about the nature of your burnout, the more effective your recovery plan will be. Let's revisit the three burnout types from earlier:

- The Overachiever's Burnout: If you identify with this type, your burnout stems from a constant drive for perfection, high expectations, and an unhealthy attachment to success and achievement. You may find yourself pushing too hard and neglecting self-care in pursuit of excellence.

- The Caregiver's Burnout: If you're constantly putting others' needs before your own and feel emotionally drained from giving too much, you likely resonate with this type. You may struggle with saying "no" and often find yourself exhausted by the demands of others.

- The Boredom Burnout: If your burnout is a result of work feeling dull or disconnected from your values, this type applies to you. You feel uninspired, lack motivation, and might be stuck in a routine that no longer brings fulfillment or meaning.

Once you've identified your burnout type, you can tailor your recovery efforts to address your unique needs. For example, an Overachiever might focus on setting realistic goals and redefining success, while a Caregiver might prioritize setting boundaries and making time for self-care.

Step 2: Reset Your Mindset About Stress and Productivity

The second step in your recovery plan involves shifting your mindset about stress and productivity. This is a critical transformation for long-term burnout prevention. Here's how to reset your perspective:

- Move from overwork to energy-based efficiency: Instead of measuring productivity by hours worked, shift to thinking about energy. It's not about how long you work but how efficiently you use your energy throughout the day. Identify activities that drain your energy and those that fuel it, and prioritize energy-restoring habits.

- Embrace progress over perfection: Release the pressure to do everything perfectly. Shift your focus toward progress-oriented thinking. Small, consistent improvements lead to more sustainable success. Perfectionism and constant hustle are often precursors to burnout, so try to celebrate the process, not just the result.

- Reframe stress as a challenge, not a threat: Rather than viewing stress as something inherently harmful, view it as an opportunity for growth. A growth mindset allows you to see challenges as experiences that can teach you something valuable, rather than feeling overwhelmed by them. This mental shift can dramatically reduce the impact of stress on your well-being.

Step 3: Rebuild Your Energy Reserves

Rebuilding your energy reserves is a key part of your recovery plan. This step combines the foundational strategies of nutrition, movement, and sleep to replenish your energy and restore balance:

- Nutrition for Energy: Implement the burnout-proof nutrition strategies from earlier. Focus on eating whole, nutrient-dense foods that stabilize your blood sugar and sustain energy throughout the day. Swap out energy-draining processed foods and prioritize meals that support long-lasting vitality. Include healthy fats, lean proteins, and complex carbohydrates to fuel your body.

- Movement for Restoration: Rather than pushing yourself to do more intense workouts, incorporate smarter movement into your routine. Focus on low-impact, energy-boosting activities that invigorate you without leaving you drained. Simple, quick bursts of exercise, like a 10-minute walk or stretching session, can do wonders for recharging your energy without overexerting yourself.

- Sleep for Recovery: Implement the sleep strategies that optimize rest and recovery. Stick to a 90-minute sleep cycle for more restorative rest. Set up a consistent wind-down routine to signal to your brain that it's time to relax. If you've been struggling with sleep, try to eliminate electronics before bed, create a peaceful environment, and focus on deep relaxation techniques that prepare you for a good night's sleep.

Putting It All Together

By following these three key steps—identifying your burnout type, resetting your mindset about stress, and rebuilding your energy reserves—you now have the framework for your Customizable Burnout Recovery Plan. The best part? You can adjust this plan as needed based on your unique challenges, lifestyle, and preferences. Here's how to start:

1. Write it Down:
   Take a moment to journal or jot down your burnout type, the mindset shifts you need to make, and the specific nutrition, movement, and sleep strategies you're going to implement. This physical act of writing out your plan will help cement your commitment to it.

2. Set Your Recovery Goals:
   Define your goals for each area—burnout type, mindset reset, and energy rebuild. What changes do you want to see? What habits will you prioritize? Make sure your goals are realistic, actionable, and aligned with your values.

3. Implement Your Plan Daily:
   Consistency is key! Make sure to revisit your plan regularly and take small daily actions to make progress. A little bit each day will add up over time, and you'll start to notice how much better you feel—

physically, emotionally, and mentally.

The Takeaway

You now have the tools to create a personalized burnout recovery plan that is built around your unique challenges and lifestyle. By identifying your burnout type, resetting your mindset, and rebuilding your energy reserves through smart nutrition, movement, and sleep, you are setting yourself up for a future that's balanced, energized, and burnout-free. This plan is customizable—meaning you can adjust it as you grow, and you can always use it to course-correct when life gets overwhelming.

Challenge: Craft Your Own Burnout Recovery Plan

1. Identify your burnout type: Reflect on whether you are an Overachiever, Caregiver, or experiencing Boredom Burnout. Write down the specific challenges that apply to you.

2. Reset your mindset: What mindset shifts will help you feel more in control and less overwhelmed? Write down the changes you need to make to move from overwork to energy-based efficiency.

3. Rebuild your energy: Create a specific action plan for nutrition, movement, and sleep that supports your recovery. What daily habits can you commit to in these areas?

By following this challenge, you will have a complete, actionable strategy for overcoming burnout and sustaining your well-being long-term.

8.2 Creating a Work-Life Balance That Actually Works for You

Work-life balance isn't a one-size-fits-all concept. It's personal, dynamic, and requires intentional choices. This section will help you create a customized work-life balance strategy that allows you to thrive, feel energized, and truly experience harmony between your personal life, work, and everything in between.

Step 4: Set Stronger Boundaries

The key to achieving balance is setting boundaries—not just at work, but in all aspects of your life. Boundaries are essential for protecting your time, energy, and mental health, especially when the demands of work, family, and other commitments can feel all-consuming.

- Protecting your time without guilt: Many people struggle with setting boundaries because they fear letting others down or feeling guilty about saying no. However, when you protect your own time, you're actually creating a space where you can show up more fully for others. Boundaries are a form of self-respect and self-care.

Here's how to set stronger boundaries:

- Be clear on your limits: Whether it's your work hours, your emotional bandwidth, or your need for personal time, define your boundaries clearly.
- Communicate your boundaries confidently: When you set a boundary, communicate it in a way that feels firm yet kind. For example, "I'm unable to take on any new tasks this week because I need to recharge and focus on my current projects."
- Honor your boundaries: Once you've set them, make sure to honor your boundaries by respecting your own needs, even if others don't fully understand or agree.

Setting boundaries can be challenging, especially if you're used to saying yes to everything. But over time, you'll start to realize that boundaries protect your energy and give you the space you need to thrive.

Step 5: Reignite Your Sense of Purpose

One of the most powerful ways to maintain balance is by reconnecting with your sense of purpose. Without a sense of purpose, work can feel draining, and life can feel like it lacks direction. It's easy to burn out when your daily actions don't align with your values or passions.

Here's how to reignite your sense of purpose:

- Align your work with your values: Start by identifying what truly matters to you—what lights you up? What drives you? Once you understand this, find ways to incorporate your values into your work and daily routines.

- Reflect on your "why": Remind yourself why you do what you do. This could be the bigger impact of your work, the values you want to share with others, or the personal satisfaction that comes with your contributions. Whether it's supporting your family, helping others, or pursuing a passion, reconnecting with your deeper "why" will help you reignite your energy and purpose.

- Make time for what fulfills you: Outside of work, focus on activities that give you joy and meaning. This could be a hobby, volunteering, or spending time with loved ones. The more you bring purpose into your life, the more energized and fulfilled you'll feel.

When you integrate a sense of purpose into both your work and personal life, you'll begin to feel more connected, motivated, and less prone to burnout. Purpose is the fuel that keeps you going, even when things get tough.

Step 6: Develop Sustainable Daily Habits

The last step in creating a work-life balance that works for you is to develop sustainable daily habits. While drastic changes might feel exciting, true balance comes from small, consistent routines that are easy to maintain over time.

Here's how to lock in powerful habits that support long-term balance:

- Start small: Begin with tiny, manageable habits that you can commit to every day. For example, if you struggle with mornings, try a 5-minute morning routine that includes stretching or journaling. If you find it hard to prioritize exercise, try taking a short walk after lunch. By starting small, you're more likely to build lasting habits.

- Habit stacking: The key to making new habits stick is pairing them with existing routines. For example, if you always have coffee in the morning, use that time to practice deep breathing for one minute. Or, after you finish your workday, make it a habit to spend 10 minutes reflecting on your day and setting your intention for tomorrow. This helps ensure your new habit becomes ingrained.

- Be consistent but flexible: The key to sustainability is consistency. Choose habits that can be easily incorporated into your daily life, but allow for flexibility when life gets busy. If something doesn't work for a while, don't abandon it—adjust it and try again.

Creating balance isn't about doing everything perfectly; it's about developing habits that nurture your well-being and support your goals. Focus on progress over perfection and embrace the small changes that lead to a more balanced, fulfilling life.

Putting It All Together

Now that you have these three steps—setting stronger boundaries, reigniting your sense of purpose, and developing sustainable habits—you're equipped to create a work-life balance that truly works for you. Balance is not about doing everything at once; it's about consciously choosing what matters most and ensuring that your time and energy are aligned with your values.

Challenge: Craft Your Work-Life Balance Plan

1. Set your boundaries: Write down the boundaries you want to set in both your personal and professional life. What are your limits when it comes to work hours, emotional energy, and personal time? Start by setting one new boundary this week and commit to honoring it.

2. Reconnect with your purpose: Take 10 minutes today to reflect on your sense of purpose. Why do you do what you do? How can you make your work more aligned with your values? Write down one small action you can take to bring more purpose into your day.

3. Create your daily habits: Choose one small habit to focus on this week that will help you create balance. Whether it's a 5-minute morning ritual, a daily movement break, or a new relaxation practice before bed, make it easy to implement and stick to it. Write down how you will incorporate it into your existing routines.

By taking action on these three steps, you will start to create a work-life balance that feels sustainable, fulfilling, and uniquely yours. Balance is not a destination—it's a journey. Keep moving forward, one small step at a time.

8.3 Your Long-Term Anti-Burnout Strategy

Burnout recovery is a dynamic, ongoing process. After putting in the effort to reset, recharge, and realign with what truly matters, it's crucial to build a strategy that supports you in the long run. The key to staying burnout-free isn't about avoiding stress altogether—it's about developing tools and habits that allow you to thrive, even when life feels chaotic.

This section is your guide to sustaining the progress you've made, ensuring that burnout stays in the rearview mirror, and creating a long-term anti-burnout strategy that works for you.

Step 7: Check In and Adjust as Needed

The first step in your long-term strategy is to regularly check in with yourself. Burnout isn't something you can cure once and forget about—it's an ongoing practice to stay aware of your mental, emotional, and physical state. Monitoring your energy and stress levels is key to preventing relapse and staying on track.

Here's how to stay proactive:

- Create a weekly check-in: Dedicate 10 minutes every week to assess your energy, stress, and overall well-being. Are there any signs of burnout creeping in? Are you feeling mentally drained or emotionally depleted? Track your mood, physical energy, and any work/life imbalances.

- Adjust when necessary: If you're noticing early signs of burnout—such as irritability, fatigue, or overwhelming stress—make the necessary adjustments. It could mean re-evaluating your boundaries, taking extra rest, or simply checking in with your goals and priorities. Flexibility is key to sustaining your progress.

Regular self-assessment ensures you stay on top of your well-being and can course-correct before burnout becomes a problem again.

How to Stay Motivated When Life Gets Busy

Life is unpredictable. Things will get hectic. Deadlines, family obligations, and other external pressures may threaten to knock you off course. The secret to maintaining progress during chaotic times is to stay motivated and committed to your self-care routine.

Here are some strategies to keep you going:

- Focus on small wins: When things feel overwhelming, shift your focus to the small, actionable steps you can take. Celebrate your wins, no matter how small. Did you get in a quick 10-minute walk today? That's a win! Did you set a boundary at work? Another win! These moments of progress help maintain momentum, even when life feels out of control.

- Prioritize your energy: When life gets busy, it's easy to slip into the habit of neglecting self-care. But that's when it's most crucial. Prioritize energy-boosting habits, like eating well, getting enough sleep, and moving your body, to keep your stress levels in check. You don't have to do everything—just focus on the key habits that support your well-being.

- Stay connected to your purpose: Revisit your "why" regularly. When you're rooted in your sense of purpose, it becomes easier to stay motivated, even in the busiest of times. Reflect on the meaningful reasons you're making these changes and stay connected to the impact your well-being has on your overall life.

Remember: Consistency is key, but it doesn't mean perfection. Life will get busy, but even the smallest effort toward maintaining your balance matters.

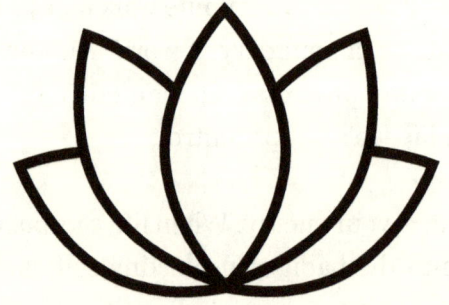

A 30-Day Burnout Recovery Challenge

Ready to implement everything you've learned? Here's a 30-Day Burnout Recovery Challenge to help you take action and start making positive changes right now. This challenge is designed to help you build sustainable habits, regain your energy, and reset your mindset, step-by-step.

Week 1: Mindset Reset

- Day 1-3: Complete your Burnout Type quiz and identify your specific burnout type.
- Day 4-7: Focus on shifting your mindset from overwork to energy-based efficiency. Try the 1% Rule to incorporate small changes that have the biggest impact.

Week 2: Boundaries and Balance

- Day 8-10: Set your first strong boundary (e.g., no emails after 6 PM).
- Day 11-14: Identify areas where you're overcommitting and practice saying "no" with grace using the scripts provided.

Week 3: Recharging and Restoring

- Day 15-17: Focus on building your energy reserves by adding small, consistent habits for nutrition, movement, and sleep.
- Day 18-21: Incorporate movement into your day using the Anti-Burnout Workout (even if it's just for 10 minutes).

Week 4: Integration and Evaluation

- Day 22-24: Try the 5-Minute Daily Practice to check in with your values and realign your actions accordingly.
- Day 25-27: Implement a daily reflection practice. Each evening, reflect on your day, and evaluate what drained your energy and what restored it.
- Day 28-30: Create your personal Burnout Recovery Plan, using the tools and strategies from this chapter.

By the end of this challenge, you will have a personalized, sustainable strategy for preventing burnout and maintaining long-term balance.

Challenge: Implement Your 30-Day Action Plan

Take out a notebook or journal and break down your 30-day Burnout Recovery Challenge into manageable tasks. You can follow the schedule above, or tailor it to your own timeline. Every few days, reflect on what's working, what needs adjustment, and celebrate every success.

The key is small, consistent actions. By following through on this 30-day plan, you'll not only reset your energy but also cultivate long-term habits that keep burnout at bay for good.

You've got this. Stay focused, stay consistent, and remember—burnout doesn't define you. Your strength, resilience, and dedication to your well-being do.

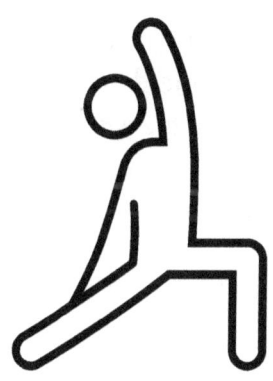

Your Path to a Burnout-Free Life

You've made it to the end of this journey, but in many ways, it's only just the beginning. The tools, strategies, and insights shared in this book aren't meant to be checked off and forgotten—they are the foundation of a life that not only survives but thrives. By taking action, even in the smallest of ways, you're already well on your way to a future of balance, fulfillment, and sustained well-being.

Key Takeaways

1. Your 7-Step System for Recovery
   Let's recap the core framework you've just explored:
   - Step 1: **Identify Your Burnout Type**—Understanding which type of burnout you're experiencing is the first step to healing.
   - Step 2: **Shift Your Mindset About Stress and Productivity**—Moving from overworking to working with energy-based efficiency.
   - Step 3: **Rebuild Your Energy Reserves**—Strategically supporting your body with nutrition, movement, and restorative sleep.
   - Step 4: **Set Stronger Boundaries**—Saying no, protecting your energy, and creating space for yourself.
   - Step 5: **Reignite Your Sense of Purpose**—Aligning your work and life with what truly matters to you.

- Step 6: **Develop Sustainable Daily Habits**—Creating habits that support long-term well-being.
- Step 7: **Check In and Adjust as Needed**—Regularly assessing your energy and stress to stay on track.

These steps provide a comprehensive roadmap to not just recover from burnout, but to build a more sustainable, fulfilling life.

> Small Changes Lead to Big Impact
> Remember, small changes are far more powerful than drastic overhauls. Consistent, incremental shifts in your habits, mindset, and daily routine will set the stage for long-term success. You don't have to overhaul your life overnight—just commit to small, manageable changes that build momentum over time. As you've seen throughout this book, it's the 1% Rule that truly works: tiny changes, compounded over time, lead to extraordinary results.
>
> Burnout Isn't a Personal Failure
> If you've been feeling overwhelmed, drained, or exhausted, know this: burnout is not a personal failure. It's a sign that something in your life needs attention. Whether it's the way you're managing stress, your lack of boundaries, or a disconnect from your purpose, burnout is a signal that your energy, time, and priorities need to be rebalanced. The good news is, you have the power to change it.

Recovery Is About Doing the Right Things in the Right Way

It's important to understand that recovery isn't about doing more. In fact, doing more can often worsen burnout. Instead, recovery is about doing the right things in the right way. Focusing on the activities that restore you, setting boundaries, managing your energy, and addressing your mindset are the foundations of true recovery. Rest and rejuvenation come from aligning with your needs—not adding more tasks to your already overloaded plate.

Small Shifts Lead to Thriving

The small shifts you make today will determine whether you stay stuck or begin to thrive. By making a commitment to your health, your energy, and your happiness now, you are setting yourself up for success—whether that means reducing stress, rediscovering purpose, or simply having more energy to enjoy your life.

I Believe In You

Now that you have the tools and knowledge to make lasting change, it's time to take action.

Pick one small habit from this book and start today. Whether it's saying no to an unnecessary commitment, incorporating a five-minute daily reflection, or prioritizing your sleep, the key is to start small and start now. Don't wait until burnout forces you to change—take control of your energy, time, and life right now.

Your future self will thank you.

You have the power to prevent burnout. By embracing small, sustainable shifts and committing to a burnout-proof life, you can thrive in all aspects of your life—without sacrificing your well-being. Take this first step and build a future that fuels your body, mind, and soul. The journey starts now.

Remember, you're not alone on this path. You've got everything you need to succeed. Here's to a future of balance, energy, and thriving—on your own terms.

Take the first step. Start now.

A Heartfelt Thank You

Thank you so much for taking the time to read this book. Your commitment to improving your life, finding balance, and preventing burnout is inspiring. By investing in yourself and your well-being, you've already made a huge step toward reclaiming your energy, your joy, and your purpose. I hope the tools and strategies shared here empower you to create lasting change and build a life that truly nourishes you.

As you move forward on this journey, remember: you don't have to do it alone. If you need help, guidance, or even just a reminder that you're on the right path, don't hesitate to reach out. Seeking support is a sign of strength, not weakness. Whether it's through community, a coach, or a trusted friend, remember that you're part of a bigger journey.

I truly wish you all the best as you take what you've learned here and apply it to your life. May you find the balance, peace, and energy you deserve.

And finally, if this book has helped you in any way, I'd be so grateful if you could take a moment to leave a review on the site where you purchased it (Amazon, for example). Your feedback not only means the world to me, but it also helps others who are searching for the same guidance and support.

For US Amazon Review:

Thank you again for your time, your trust, and your commitment to becoming the best version of yourself.

With gratitude and best wishes,

Andrea Sinclair

A Reminder

Please don't forget that as a token of my appreciation and a way of saying thanks for your purchase, I'm offering the short book **Sleep Your Way to Balance: Nighttime Rituals to Recharge Your Body and Mind** for FREE to my readers.

To get instant access scan the QR code or just go to:

https://andreasinclairbooks.com/free-gift

Inside the book, you will discover:

- Nighttime Rituals to Recharge
- Science-backed Tips and Tricks
- 30 Minute Wind Down Formula

If you want to improve your sleep and feel better, make sure to grab the free book!

Resources

American Psychological Association. (n.d.). Stress in America: The State of Stress in America. https://www.apa.org/news/stress

Brené Brown. (2018). Dare to Lead: Brave work. Tough conversations. Whole hearts. Random House.

Chopra, D. (2019). The Healing Self: A Revolutionary New Plan to Supercharge Your Immunity and Stay Well for Life. Harmony.

Center for Humane Technology. (n.d.). About Us. https://www.humanetech.com

Goleman, D. (2006). Emotional Intelligence: Why It Can Matter More Than IQ. Bantam.

Grant, A. (2013). Give and Take: A Revolutionary Approach to Success. Viking.

Greenfield, S. (2020). Mind Change: How Digital Technologies Are Leaving Their Mark on Our Brains. Random House.

Hallowell, E. M. (2005). Driven to Distraction: Recognizing and Coping with Attention Deficit

Disorder. Anchor Books.

Harvard Health Publishing. (2020). The Power of Sleep: What Happens During Sleep and How to Get Better Rest. https://www.health.harvard.edu/staying-healthy/the-power-of-sleep

Kabat-Zinn, J. (2005). Wherever You Go, There You Are: Mindfulness Meditation in Everyday Life. Hyperion.

Mayo Clinic. (2020). Burnout: Symptoms and Causes. https://www.mayoclinic.org/diseases-conditions/burnout/symptoms-causes/syc-20310072

McGonigal, K. (2015). The Upside of Stress: Why Stress Is Good for You, and How to Get Good at It. Avery.

Mindful. (2021). How to Practice Mindfulness. https://www.mindful.org/what-is-mindfulness/

Psychology Today. (2020). How to Recognize and Prevent Burnout. https://www.psychologytoday.com/us/blog/the-clarity/202002/how-recognize-and-prevent-burnout

Sweeney, L. (2019). The Art of Saying No: How to Set Boundaries and Prioritize Your Well-Being.
Hachette Books.

How to Pivot from Burnout to Balance

www.ingramcontent.com/pod-product-compliance
Lightning Source LLC
Chambersburg PA
CBHW031154020426
42333CB00013B/656